LOSE WEIGHT, GET HEALTHY

...and <u>NEVER</u> Have to Be on a Diet Again!

Nutrition & Health Information, Eating Plan,
Recipes, and Lifestyle Guidelines for
Becoming the Healthiest Person You Can Be

By Nancy Addison

Organic Healthy Lifestyle Publishing

Lose Weight, Get Healthy ...And Never Have to Be on a Diet Again: Nutrition & Health Information, Eating Plan, Recipes, and Lifestyle Guidelines for Becoming the Healthiest Person You Can Be

Published by Organic Healthy Lifestyle Publishing.
ISBN-10: 1517760712
ISBN-13: 978-1517760717

Nancy Alisa Gibbons Addison
Nancy@OrganicHealthyLifestyle.com
www.OrganicHealthyLifestyle.com

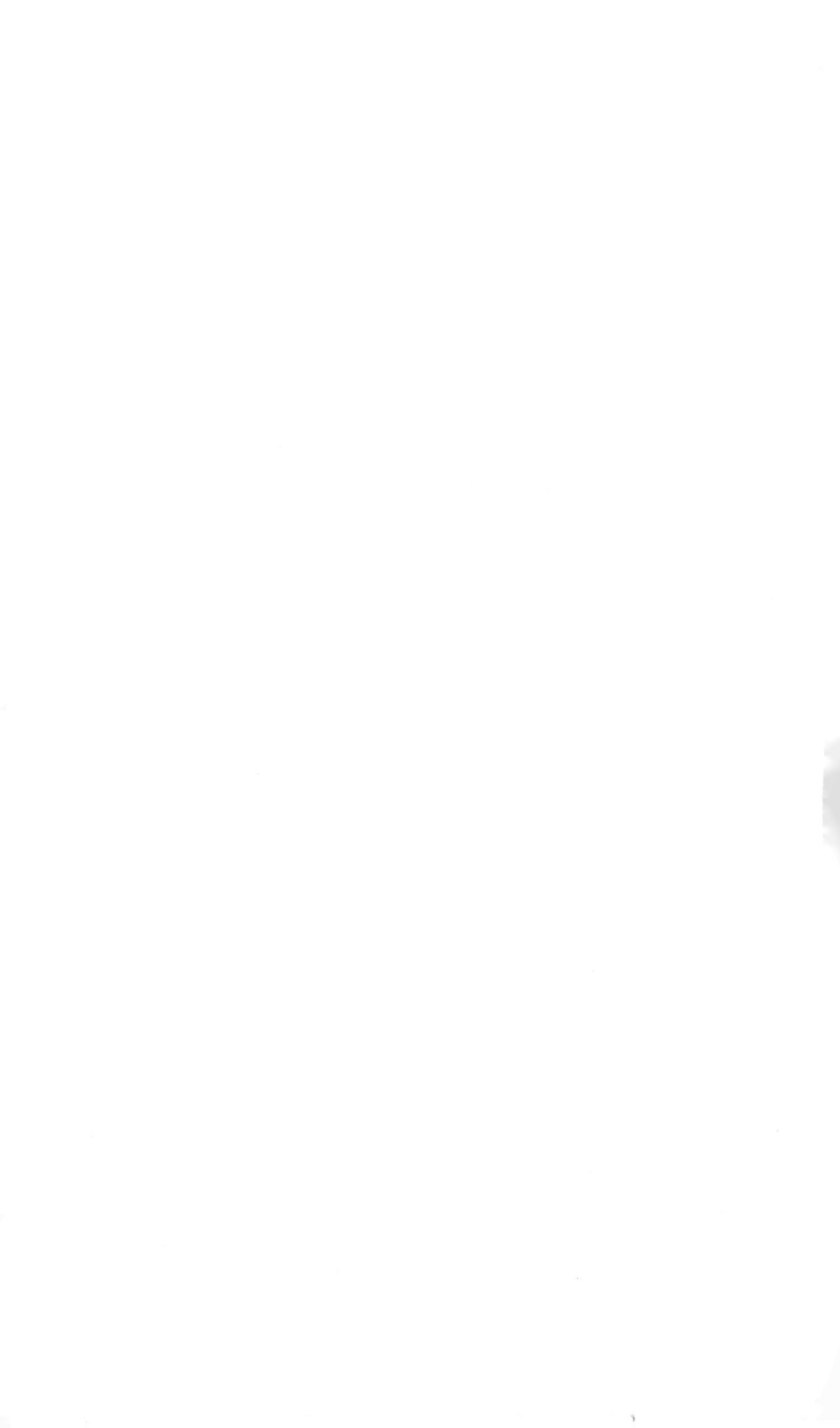

Contents

Foreword

Nancy's book is a work of art. She takes very complicated, well-researched information and makes it easy to read. It is a great resource for both medical professionals as well as the lay person.

The genius of this book is that she has combined the best of all the current, leading-edge research, digested it, and given it back in scrumptious, easy-to-make recipes. Something delicious for all palates!

It is a realistic approach to healthy weight loss. I highly recommend this book to anyone who wishes to lose weight, get healthy, and never have to be on a diet again.

Nancy has made losing weight practical and beautifully simple.

Dr. Sandra Bontemps

Dr. Sandra Bontemps is a Palm Beach Chiropractor by licensure. Her North Palm Beach practice combines Neuro Emotional Technique (NET), Total Body Modification (TBM), Acupuncture, Craniosacral Therapy, Chiropractic, Applied Kinesiology, Homeopathy, and Nutrition.

Introduction

B ecoming a healthier person, for most, is an exciting adventure! But, many of my friends and children's friends have tried to become healthier and lose weight, only to find they would gain weight quickly after they stopped their diets. They soon found themselves on a constant diet roller coaster, losing muscle as well as fat, then eventually regaining fat that was even harder to lose the next time around. Rather than swinging through various diets, it is more important and sustainable to develop a healthy lifestyle that works best for you. My friends simply didn't know how to be the healthiest people they could be. This includes not only what to eat or what not to eat, but also how to maintain an active and wholesome lifestyle. This book will enable you to reach and maintain your weight loss and health goals simply and successfully.

In this book, I will guide you through the necessary nutrition information, lifestyle changes, and suggestions. I will give you tips for eating out and traveling, and share daily menu examples. I will give you some basic yet delicious recipes I have developed since I became a thinner and healthier person.

My own journey began in 1987. I was a bit bewildered at first about what to eat and what to feed my children. Through trial and error and years of research, I found this lifestyle and diet to be progressively easier to maintain as time went on. People today are more aware and concerned with the wholesomeness of their food than ever before. Times are changing, and today there are many healthier choices at grocery stores and at most restaurants than when I was starting out in Dallas, Texas. Healthy, organic, and local foods are more accessible to us than they were twenty-seven years ago.

Despite this very positive shift, there are still many ingredients to be aware of and to look out for. Reading this book will help you, and enable you to begin your own journey towards better health and awareness of the foods you eat. It will also ensure that your health and weight loss goals are not only met, but also maintained. You can do this! Adventures in food await you!

1
Lifestyle Challenges

Sometimes when we make a lifestyle change, other people see it as threatening, because it makes them question how they themselves are living. This is a challenge, particularly if you are trying to change your eating and lifestyle habits, while your family and friends have not decided to make this change. Throughout your own quest for health, remember to be strong, hang in there, and stick with your program and the commitments you have made to yourself.

Your friends and family will soon begin to see you losing weight, getting healthier, and feeling better. They may ask you how you are doing this. When this happens, simply explain what foods you do or do not eat. Explain that you are making a lifestyle change to live a longer, happier, and healthier life. From my experience, educating people in a kind and informative manner is often very effective. I believe people mean well, but often lack the proper knowledge. With the right information, you can help the people you love become healthier and happier, too. Doing it by example is an excellent way to get those you love on board. Then you have a great support group for everyone.

I try not to push my way of thinking on others. I believe one of the best ways to bring about change is from within, and by leading my life as I feel is best. Thus, I live as an example of what I believe to be true, and I find I bring about more positive change that way. People around me are not faced with a miserable complainer, lecturer, or self-righteous preacher they want to avoid, but rather a person who lives by what she believes, and who brings a little variety to the occasion. Over the years, I have learned to deal with food situations in a savvier and more flexible way than I may have when I was younger.

The other day, I was put in charge of making macaroni and cheese for a dinner party. The dinner party hostess was apprehensive. I used organic, whole-grain pasta and flour, coconut oil, and some other alternative ingredients that I thought would be healthier. I also used rennet-free, organic cheeses from a farmer I know who raises his animals in a truly cruelty-free way. The cheeses were free of harmful additives, such as hormones and antibiotics.

Everyone loved my mac and cheese! This was a group of dinner party guests who do not normally eat this way. In fact, they didn't really care, or even know, whether the grains were whole or not. They did not know if the milk I used was cow's, goat's, almond, rice, oat, organic, cruelty-free, or not. I didn't tell them the milk I used was made of rice, with no dairy in it at all. And honestly, I don't think they could even tell! Just by doing this, I may have made a little headway in sharing my vision of a healthier pasta dish.

On another occasion, I made nut cheese for the cheese dish I was asked to bring somewhere. It was received well and with curiosity. I am not sure I converted anyone to my way of eating, but I did enlighten some to the fact that you can make a pretty tasty dairy-free cheese, that is actually from nuts.

Begin your journey by having faith and trying the various healthier diet choices that your heart tells you to try, and see how that works. Some people's diet choices may change over time with age, environment, lifestyle, and circumstance. Balance and flexibility can make life much more enjoyable. For example, I found I needed to have a little extra flexibility when I travel to foreign countries. I won't always have everything exactly as I would like it.

Some people, who have everything "set in stone" about how they are going to eat or live, run into situations or circumstances that are difficult and challenging to their diets. Unfortunately, they fall apart when things don't go exactly as they planned or wanted. Balance, flexibility, and the ability to live in the moment can be the difference between success and failure, joy and anger, and satisfaction and frustration. Live in the moment, be present, listen to your heart, and try to do the best and right thing for you and your body at the time. Life is just that: personal choices.

Find what works best for you by listening to your heart and your own body. You are the best guide and judge of your body and your health. This book will help you to make the optimal choices of foods for you. For many of us in transition, be it with new food choices or with life in general, it takes baby steps. Becoming a healthier person is a journey. Simply start the journey, and see where it takes you!

2
Lifestyle Suggestions:
Thoughts on Eating Plan and
Exercise

The first part of your weight loss program should focus primarily on vegetarian foods. There will be a few non-vegetarian meals to choose from. But, if you are really serious about losing weight and getting healthier, then cutting down on meat, chicken, or fish-based foods is the optimal way to begin. To jumpstart your weight loss, it is also important to begin by cutting out wheat and corn. Focus instead on eating whole foods and avoiding all boxed and packaged foods, which are often highly processed and filled with preservatives.

For the first two weeks, I recommend completely omitting meat, chicken, fish, dairy, corn, and wheat. After your body has lightly detoxed, you can begin slowly adding a few healthier chicken and fish dishes back into your diet. If you can completely eliminate corn and wheat from your diet, your health will greatly benefit. It feels overwhelming at first, but it will become easier as you learn to do it. You should also increase your intake of fresh and organic fruits, vegetables, whole grains, and living raw foods. I will elaborate on this later.

This lifestyle plan also involves getting yourself moving. Exercise is important for everyone and is necessary to keep your body healthy. We need to move! If you can't stand up, then move while seated. Exercise your arms and upper body, if that is all you can do at the moment. For example, while sitting at your desk or sitting in the car, stretch your arms. Stretch and move as much as possible. If you can move more than that, then do what you can or what best fits your body for at least 30 minutes per day, four times per week. Those who can walk, should walk for a minimum of 30 minutes per day (or at least four times per week), preferably in a brisk manner.

Studies show that when you exercise before breakfast, it stabilizes your blood sugar immediately and energizes you for the rest of the day. Studies show people who exercise before breakfast lose weight quicker.

Also, if you add short bursts of high intensity to your workout, it can increase your fat burn by up to 36%. So, what does that look like? If you are walking, add a minute or two of jogging to your walk. If you are on a treadmill, add a minute or two of a faster, more intense pace to the workout intermittently. It is so easy to do, and, *wow*, what a difference it can make! Try picking up a new fun form of exercise, such as dance classes or yoga. Anything to get your body moving!

When you feel ready, increase your exercise time to 40–60 minutes every day. Increase and expand your exercise routine, as you feel able. If you miss a day, don't get upset with yourself. Simply get back to your routine again tomorrow. Always be kind to yourself. Just pick up where you left off and get going again. Ideally, we should exercise every single day, even if it's something as basic as walking. Getting the body oxygenated and the circulatory system going is important to maintaining an active metabolism. It is also very helpful to our overall health and wellbeing.

In addition, start doing more weight training! It doesn't have to be much or too heavy. Find what works for you. Weight training increases bone density, and it improves muscle mass, balance, and connective tissue strength. It also increases your metabolism!

Weight training should be a priority if you really want to burn more fat. Lifting weights raises your metabolism long after you finish working out. It is estimated that your metabolism can stay elevated up to 39 hours afterwards! As you build more muscle, muscle is more metabolically active than fat. Some estimate that each extra pound of muscle you gain burns 30 or more extra calories a day. It's estimated that a pound of muscle burns six calories at rest, compared to two calories burned by a pound of fat.

If you commit to this lifestyle (regular exercise, some weightlifting, and wholesome foods) and diet (completely vegetarian or vegan, gluten-free and mostly living, raw food), you can lose anywhere between 5 and 15 pounds per week. It depends on you!

As we move into a new lifestyle, consider the following tips. They are easy to do, and they are important adjustments that will really help you live a healthier life.

Always eat sitting down at some form of table. This does not mean eating in the car. In fact, a good lifestyle means to never eat in your car, standing up, walking, or in front of the refrigerator. If you are hungry and standing at the refrigerator, pull up a chair! Really! No, just kidding—but really, don't stand at the refrigerator and eat! Instead, simply take something out, put it on a small plate, and then sit down at the table to eat your food slowly and mindfully. Enjoy each bite, and chew your food thoroughly. Savor your food and enjoy it. Make it an experience that is fun, enjoyable, and relaxing.

My daughter, Amanda, put a note on her refrigerator door that says, "Nothing tastes as good as skinny feels." It was a reminder of her goals. I think it is a good reminder and may help stop the temporary urge to mindlessly eat food for whatever reason.

Avoid mindless eating in front of the TV. Turn off the television and focus on what you are doing. You are nourishing your body and enjoying your meal. Light a candle, turn on some music and sit down and eat in a relaxing manner. When chewed properly, your food should be liquid by the time you swallow it. What this means is, stop eating fast food, and stop eating food fast. Food that comes through your car window is probably not the healthiest food, and it won't help you to lose weight. If you are serious about losing weight, then this is a key to your healthy weight loss and healthy lifestyle.

Chew your food completely without washing it down with liquids. In other words, do not drink liquids with your meals. When we are eating our meals, the most important thing is to digest our food completely, absorb the nutrients, and get the waste out of our body as efficiently as possible. When we drink liquids with our food, we are watering down our digestive juices in our stomach, and the food is not as effectively digested. We also may not chew our food as thoroughly if we wash it down with a liquid. So, try to avoid liquids with your meals. Chew your food as completely as possible, until it is almost liquid by the time you swallow it. Only have liquid there if you need it.

This is an important part of losing weight, sustaining efficient digestion, and having more optimum health.

Slowing down when we eat may be an unfamiliar lifestyle change, but it is incredibly valuable for health. So, slow down. Eat your food slowly, enjoy your food, and chew it up completely. Studies show that when people eat slowly and completely, they eat less, are more satisfied, and have a healthier weight.

I was once eating lunch with my friend, who struggles with her weight. She was having a fairly healthy salad and a diet soda. As she talked, I watched her gulp down her salad and wash it down with her soda. I realized it didn't matter what she was eating. She was watering down her digestive juices, not chewing her food properly, and shutting down her digestive system with the ice in her drink. Ice in our drinks shocks our digestive systems, freezing it for an hour and a half. No matter what my friend was eating, it was not being digested well, which prevented her from getting the necessary nutrients from it. These are all factors which contribute to a person's being overweight.

Diet soda also contains many addictive chemicals which make you gain weight and dehydrate your body. Cutting out any kind of soda, especially diet sodas, is imperative to losing weight and improving your health.

As an added guideline, try to eat for 15 minutes, and then pause for 10 minutes before resuming your meal. This is especially helpful for preventing overeating, which also slows your digestive system and leads to weight gain. This doesn't mean drinking something or checking your email during that time. Instead, just sit, talk, or listen to music and relax. This gives your body time to begin to digest your food. This break also gives your mind the time to recognize when your stomach is full. This way, you will eat less without feeling deprived. This is a key element to losing weight or staying slim, without deprivation.

An additional fun fact: For some reason, blue plates make us eat less. By using blue plates for dining, we play a small psychological trick on ourselves, so we actually eat less.

Eat three good meals a day with little or no snacking. Eating a healthy breakfast and lunch is an important key to health. Don't nibble here and there. Snacking can add up quickly without your even noticing how much you actually eat. Small snacks can also make your body dependent upon constant nourishment. Why would your body consume unwanted extra weight if it is never hungry, because it is always being filled up? You need to give your body a reason to burn off that weight. Get your food out, prepare your meal, and put it on a small plate. Sit down and take time to chew your food well. Savor your meals, relax, and enjoy.

Consuming a light dinner is preferable. Eat your larger meals during the day, and keep your dinner lighter. You don't want your body working all night digesting food, when it is meant to be sleeping and resting.

Spacing meals allows ample time to have our water or liquids in between, without watering down our digestive juices. For optimal digestion, wait two hours after a meal to drink water or liquids. Try to drink most of the water you need for the day in that space between meals.

Drink half your body weight (in pounds) in ounces of water per day. This means if you are 100 pounds, you would drink 50 ounces of water every day. Quality water is important. Water is a unique element. According to my research, water should have electrolytes and be free of chlorine and fluoride. This not only increases the health properties of water, but also allows for better absorption into our bodies. Water is important to life. More than 66% of our body is water. Everyone needs to stay hydrated every single day by drinking high-quality water. This may be one of the most important things we can do for the health of our body.

The best time to have water is the first thing in the morning when we wake up. This starts the hydration process immediately. Whatever we put into our body first will be absorbed like a sponge, so this is the ideal time to have a large glass of water. It is widely known that many diseases are caused by cellular dehydration. Therefore, it is imperative to stay hydrated in order to avoid disease. Even in the winter, when we may not feel like we need to drink as much water, we need to stay just as hydrated as we do in the summer.

Our body needs the naturally occurring minerals in water to absorb it and be properly hydrated. Real, natural water has minerals in it. Most of the water we drink today has been purified. When water is purified, the purification process depletes the water of all the minerals. These minerals are also known as electrolytes. When we drink water that has been depleted of its minerals, essential minerals are pulled from stored areas in our bodies in order to process the water.

At the Tree of Life, Dr. Gabriel Cousens has a sign above the water cooler saying to add sea salt to the water. At his retreat center, he uses a reverse osmosis water purification system, one of the best water purification systems there is. But, while it does remove all the bad chemicals we *don't* want in our water, it also removes all of the good minerals we *do* want in our water. Next to his water, he keeps little jars of whole sea salt to add to your water when filling your glass. This way, you add the minerals back into your water, so you do not have to pull important minerals from your body to process it. By simply adding a pinch or two of whole sea salt to your water before drinking it, you replace the natural minerals (electrolytes) that have been removed during the purification process. This allows your body to hydrate in the most effective way.

We need to drink enough water in a day to really hydrate our body. Between meals is the best time to do that. So, have your water about two and a half hours after a meal, or an hour before your meal. Coffee, alcoholic drinks, and sodas are not hydrating and do not count. In fact, you will need to drink extra water to make up for the dehydrating effects caused by consuming these beverages. Freshly juiced vegetable or fruit juices are hydrating, but you need to drink them within 20 minutes of being juiced in order to get the full nutritional benefits.

Hunger pangs can be signs of dehydration. So, consuming the proper amount of high-quality water at the right times throughout the day is very important.

Cut wheat and corn out of your diet. Wheat and corn should be greatly reduced or completely eliminated from your diet. Wheat has the unusual characteristic of being able to raise blood sugar rapidly. Additionally, due to today's genetic modification of wheat, it now contains up to 80%

more gluten than it did 100 years ago. Gluten is the glue-like substance that is part of various grains. When we eat wheat or other grains that contain gluten (and are refined, highly processed, or have had the fiber removed), it is quite literally like eating glue. If you do choose to eat it, eat organic and whole grain varieties.

Corn is not only high in sugar, but also prone to molds and funguses that can be toxic to us and compromise our immune systems. Most corn today is grown as a genetically modified food, which has a Bt toxin built into it. Studies show this toxin can eat holes in the stomach and intestinal tract, which causes leaky gut, gluten intolerance, and many other health problems. This Bt toxin is in many GMO (genetically modified) foods, such as soy.[1]

You will be surprised at how much better you will feel and how much weight you will lose when you cut these two foods from your diet. Be sure to read ingredient labels, because corn, soy, and wheat are used in almost all processed foods in one form or another. Become a savvy ingredient label reader! Your body will love you for it!

Clean Your Fruits and Vegetables. Clean all fruits and vegetables well. This not only removes unwanted bacteria, but also unnatural toxins such as pesticides and preservatives. An inexpensive way to clean fruits and vegetables is to soak them in a mixture of unfiltered apple cider vinegar or food-grade hydrogen peroxide and water for about 15–20 minutes. Use one tablespoon apple cider vinegar or peroxide to one gallon water, or ¼ cup for a sink full of water.

3
Cleanse Your Body

There are many reasons to clean out the inside of the body on a regular basis. Clean cells and a clean body, inside and out, are the secrets to having more energy, looking younger, and having a stronger immune system.

We *need* to cleanse because we acquire toxins in our bodies on a regular basis. We live in a world that is literally saturated with toxins. We can get toxins by breathing in polluted air, taking showers in chlorinated tap water, drinking tap water, and eating foods when we don't know their source or preparation method. Additionally, our bodies become acidic through stress and the foods we eat. These toxins and acids hurt our bodies deep within our cells. How can the body have a clean liver, blood, or lymphatic system if it is filled with toxins, acid, and waste? A clean intestinal system and frequent, thorough bowel movements are key factors of a truly healthful system.

We absorb most of our nutrients though the intestinal wall. If it is clean, we are able to absorb the nutrients. If it is not clean but is instead full of waste and rancid debris, then the body won't get the nutrients it needs. Dr. Anthony Bassler, a gastroenterologist, said, "Every physician should realize the intestinal toxemias (poisons) are the most important primary and contributing cause of many disorders and diseases of the body."[2]

We also need to cleanse because our intestines can become thick with plaque over time. This "mucoid plaque" can result from consuming foods like milk, wheat, and meat. It can be thick and rubbery. It can even look a little like a rope when it exits the body.

In the book *Tissue Cleansing through Bowel Management*, Dr. Bernard Jensen, DC, ND, PhD addresses this:

> The heavy mucus coating in the colon thickens and becomes a host of putrefaction. The blood capillaries to the colon begin to pick up the toxins, poisons, and noxious debris as it seeps through the bowel wall. All tissues and organs of the body are now taking on toxic substances. Here is the beginning of true autointoxication on a physiological level. One autopsy revealed a colon to be nine inches in diameter with a passage through it no larger than a pencil. The rest was caked up layer upon layer of encrusted fecal material. This accumulation can have the consistency of truck tire rubber. It's that hard and black. Another autopsy revealed a stagnant colon to weigh in at an incredible 40 pounds.[3]

Dr. Richard Anderson, ND, NMD addresses the subject of plaque as well. Dr. Anderson, an expert on colon cleansing, wrote *Cleanse and Purify Thyself, Volumes 1 & 2.* In an article on colon plaque, he says:

> The phrase, "mucoid plaque" is a coined term that I use to describe various conditions found throughout the body, especially in hollow organs and the alimentary canal. It is a substance that the body naturally creates under unnatural conditions, such as attacks from acids, drugs, heavy metals, and toxic chemicals.[4]

Professional cleanses, like colonics or enemas, can get this old, leftover waste and plaque out of the intestinal tract. (See "Colonic Cleanse," below.)

I recommend cleansing for a minimum of three days and as long as 21 days to detoxify the body and adjust its pH on a regular basis. This will keep the inner environment of the body's digestive system cleaner, healthier, and able to support a healthy immune system. Along with this comes an additional benefit. A major part of the body's happiness chemical, serotonin, is synthesized in the gastrointestinal tract. It is no wonder people feel happier and better when their bowels are clean and functioning in the optimum way! I do a month-long cleanse every January to start off the New Year fresh and renewed after too much holiday party munching.

Each time you cleanse, it will get easier. Eventually, or maybe very quickly, you will see a difference in how you feel. You will have to make a personal decision about the length of your cleanse. Many physicians think 21 days is the best length. You may want to consult your physician before starting a cleanse, or do the cleanse under his or her guidance. Many wonderful physicians and clinics have juice fasts, cleanses, and other programs you can do under their guidance.

Garden of Life makes a nice, easy cleanse. But for those who wish to create their own cleanse, here are a few different types I have used and found very effective.

High-Fiber Cleanse

This is a basic cleanse I have been doing for more than 25 years. I raised my children on it. The two things I think are most lacking in the American diet are good, healthy fiber and good, healthy green foods. This cleanse has both. Quite simply, it is made up of the good, healthy food that most people lack in their normal, everyday diet.

The nutrients will feed your body as well as help flush and pull toxins and acids out of the cells. The fiber will absorb these toxins and expand like a sponge. You will then drink a lot of water, which will create a cleaning effect. Along with the sponge-like fiber, the toxic particles, plaque, and other debris that might be lodged in the intestines will be dragged out. Each time you cleanse, it will clean out a little more. Think of the layers of an onion. When you start, you will get one layer, and the next time, you will get the next layer.

This cleanse is done morning, noon, and night for 3–14 days or more. You may eventually find this is a good part of your daily or weekly routine. I do this cleanse a few times a week, year-round, as a normal part of my diet.

You can buy the ingredients for this cleanse at most health food stores or grocery stores. It calls for raw organic green food powder. But, when possible, I use fresh, organic green barley grass or wheat grass juice instead of the powder. Fresh is always best, but the concentrated, powdered form makes this cleanse easy to use anytime and anywhere. If you have trouble drinking green, powdery, high-fiber drinks, buy the green food powder in capsule form.

This cleanse also calls for psyllium husks. They expand very quickly when put into water and will turn into a thick clump you cannot drink. So, either take psyllium husks in capsule form or drink it quickly once you add water to it. The psyllium husks will then expand in your stomach, which is why you are taking them. They are a great fiber which makes you feel full as it works like a large sponge to clean out your body's organs on its way through. By absorbing toxins, it is able to pull them, as well as waste, from your body.

A kalenite pill is another key ingredient of this cleanse. Kalenite is a blend of eight herbs "known for their ability to support proper elimination through the colon, liver, kidneys, and lymphatic system, as well as helping to tone these organs of elimination so they can function more efficiently."[5] It pulls toxins from your cells naturally and prevents you from feeling queasy. Pumpkin seeds are optional, but they work really well if you have parasites. Chia seeds add anti-inflammatory, essential Omega 3 fatty acids.

Note: This is my favorite cleanse, but it is only for someone who is able to have regular bowel movements. If you are not having regular bowel movements, then you may need to simply consume raw fresh vegetable juice three times per day, or do colonics, until your bowel movements are regular.

Ingredients:
concentrated raw organic green food powder (or capsules, or fresh organic barley grass or wheatgrass juice)
organic psyllium husks
freshly ground, fresh, organic, raw pumpkin seeds (optional)
kalenite pills
probiotic capsules
digestive enzymes

Directions:

Days 1–3

For one to three full days, three or four times a day, starting first thing in the morning, drink an eight-ounce glass of mineral-rich water, coconut water, or ginger root juice along with:

- 2-3 tsp. concentrated raw organic green food powder (or 8–10 capsules)
- 1 tsp. organic psyllium husks (3 capsules)

If you are using freshly juiced greens, drink 6–8 ounces of the juice with the psyllium husks.

Throughout the day, drink a couple of liters (one ounce of water for every two pounds of your body weight) of mineral-rich water, coconut water, fresh ginger root juice, and more fresh, organic, vegetable juices throughout the day.

Days 2–21

Starting on the second, third, or fourth day, depending on how long you are able to go with only liquids, mix together:

- 1 tsp. concentrated raw organic green food powder (or 8–10 capsules, or 6–8 ounces of fresh organic barley grass, or wheat grass juice)
- 1 tsp. organic psyllium husks
- ½ tsp. freshly ground, fresh, organic, raw pumpkin seeds (optional)
- 4 oz. purified water

Drink it very quickly with:
- 1 kalenite pill
- 1 probiotic capsule
- 1 digestive enzyme

Immediately afterward, drink a mixture of:
- 18 oz. pure water
- 1/8 tsp. high-quality sea salt.

Drink as much high-quality water throughout the day as you can (one ounce of water for every two pounds of your body weight). This is very important for helping flush the toxins out of the body.

Do this every day for 3–14 days minimum. If you are really serious about this, you can do it for 21 days. Start first thing in the morning on an empty stomach, and repeat at lunch and dinner (before 6 p.m.).

Please Note: You will go to the bathroom a few hours after you do the High-Fiber Cleanse. Feeling unwell is a symptom of a large amount of toxins being eliminated from the body. It means you need to drink a lot of water to help flush out all of the toxins and assist the fiber in continuing its journey out of your body.

All food should be efficiently digested, its nutrients absorbed, and its waste eliminated. If you are eating three times per day, then you should be having bowel movements three times per day. The more fiber you ingest, the easier and more efficiently the waste will be eliminated. There is not a set time period for this, but ideally it should be anywhere from 3–12 hours after each meal. You can test your digestive function by eating a meal of raw or slightly steamed red beets. The deep red color in the bowel movement will allow you to see when that meal is eliminated. This is an easy way to see if your body is eliminating quickly and efficiently.

If you are not having regular bowel movements, then don't include the psyllium husks in your cleanse until you are. If you have already started the cleanse and are not having regular bowel movements, then stop the psyllium husks immediately and take only the greens until you are going regularly. If you feel uncomfortable and are not having bowel movements, you may want to get a colonic series to help get your system cleaned out and moving again.

Drink lots of water, fresh green organic vegetable juices, and other liquids to keep the toxins, acid, and waste moving out of the body. This is so important! This cleanse is cleaning out the inside of your body. With the removal of the plaque, waste, and debris, you will also be alkalizing your body and helping your body maintain a healthier pH. Greens are highly alkalizing.

This may seem like a lot of work, but each time you do it, it will get easier, and you will start to feel better and have more energy! In situations where you feel you must have some food or really need something to chew, you can eat snacks or meals consisting of raw or lightly steamed organic vegetables about an hour before or after consuming the cleanse. You may also chew on celery sticks or cucumber slices. You may sprinkle pure whole sea salt and chia seeds on your food. If you feel you must use some fat, then try using a little bit of coconut oil. The coconut oil can give you additional nourishment as well as energy.

Colonic Cleanse

If your body is not eliminating wastes efficiently after each meal, there may be some blockage in the intestinal tract. Anyone who has been a meat eater or a consumer of processed foods, fried foods, and trans fats may have blockages, plaque, or debris lodged in the colon. After years and years of eating meals that are not completely digested or moved out of the body, layers and layers of waste build up. Natalia Rose, a New York clinical nutritionist, says that if you wake up in the morning, have a bowel movement, pull in your gut, and it is almost to your spine, then you have an empty and clean intestine. If you cannot do this, then your intestines are full of undigested waste stuck in the tissues like cement.

Master colon therapist Gil Jacobs explains that a laxative will do nothing for the normal person who is eating fairly well, except release the very newest waste, and then drive the older waste deeper into the tissue and make it harder to remove. The laxative will irritate the bowels. He and Natalia Rose believe in colonic cleansing and recommend the gravity method. The client reclines in a large chair, and a small quantity of warm water is very slowly introduced into the colon by a narrow tube. Then the water runs out of the colon, being released to flow out through a tube and directly into the plumbing. The hydrotherapist answers questions, guiding or assisting whenever needed. Having a colonic is actually very easy. The water cleanses the walls of the intestine. Each time a colonic is done, another layer of plaque or waste can be washed out of the lining of the colon.

People say, "I got a colonoscopy, and it was fine." However, a colonoscopy doesn't clean out the colon. It doesn't pull out the toxins or plaque embedded in the lining of the intestines. It is like a bullet going through the barrel of a gun. On the other hand, a colonic actually washes out the debris, plaque, and whatever else is stuck in the layers of the intestinal wall.

Colonics are recommended for people with a high degree of inflammation, constipation, and/or plaque in their colon. Some people find it so useful that they continue to do it once a month or more just to stay clean. Gil and Natalia say that a person who grew up eating a standard American diet of bread, meat, trans fats, sugar, and junk food could get a colonic every week for the rest of his or her life and still not have all of the waste completely removed from the colon.

A raw food diet will help awaken the body and the waste, and help get it to move out. Changing your diet to mostly raw food will help, because the food is more likely to be completely or close to completely digested. Your body will start to cleanse itself of toxins because of the antioxidant-rich food and fiber. When the colon and the rest of the intestinal tract are cleaned up and running free and clear, the whole body will start to work in harmony. Many people will find their joint problems, headaches, back aches, skin problems, and hair problems simply disappear when they finally get their colon and intestines clean and oxygenated.

Natalia Rose also recommends enemas as another way to remove waste from the bowels. They can work well and get waste to come out of the tissues. Gil and Natalia also recommend putting a small step stool in front of the toilet. If you put your feet on the small stool when using the toilet, your intestinal tract has a better curve, making it much easier to move waste through the tract.

Coffee Enema

The liver and gallbladder can get overloaded with toxins. When this happens, a coffee enema can be the solution. Coffee enemas are used to increase the liver's detoxification capacity. The coffee enema was a staple of the Merck Manual (considered the "bible" of medical books) until it was removed fairly recently. It wasn't removed because it didn't work—because the coffee enema has been proven to work—but it was removed. Many of the extremely successful natural cancer centers use the coffee enema as a staple of their health programs. In fact, it is a required part of the Gerson Therapy program.

In an intense health program with juicing, the juices begin nourishing the body. The high antioxidant levels force cells to release toxins into the bloodstream. This can put a burden or toxin overload on the liver. The liver alone, especially in a cancer patient, cannot handle the sudden flood of toxins being released into the bloodstream. Coffee enemas help flush the toxins from the toxin-saturated liver. This helps the liver regain the ability to flush even more toxins from the blood stream.

Colonics have the same purpose as the coffee enema. Colonics cleanse the bowel. Coffee enemas increase the liver's detoxification volume. Substances in coffee stimulate a main detoxification enzyme in the liver and dilate the bile ducts to increase the flow of bile.

Another benefit of the coffee enema is help emptying the bowel. It would be wise to make certain you are free of constipation before attempting a coffee enema. A series of colonics would encourage a cleaner bowel and make the coffee enema more effective. Avoid doing both together in the same day. This can be depleting to your body. You can read more about coffee enemas on the Gerson Therapy website, Gerson.org.

This enema requires a particular type of coffee. One highly recommended brand is S. A. Wilson's *Gold Roast* from SAWilsons.com. You can order an enema kit, including instructions, from the Optimum Health Institute.

Oil Pulling

Oil pulling is an Ayurvedic Remedy used to enhance oral health and well-being. Oil pulling detoxifies the body, removes unsightly stains on teeth, and prevents illness and disease.

My daughter and I did it infrequently for a while and never noticed a difference; but when we did it on a continual basis for 15 days without interruption, the difference was noticeable. Amanda saw a huge difference in her health, gums, teeth, and how she felt when she finally did it consistently. I have noticed a significant difference between when I do it and when I don't. When I do this in the morning, my mouth seems amazingly clean and fresh. So, I recommend doing it on a consistent basis, if you are going to try it.

Ingredients:
Pure, organic coconut oil
Unrefined sea salt
Tongue scraper Toothbrush
Purified, (non-chlorinated) water

Directions:
First thing in the morning, before brushing your teeth or eating anything, take 1 teaspoon of pure, organic coconut oil into your mouth and swish the oil in your mouth, tilting your head back, so that it can get to the back molars. (It may taste weird the first few days, but you will get used to it—if you stick with it.) It is very important that you keep the oil in your mouth the whole time and **Avoid Swallowing It**.

You suck and pull the oil through your teeth and chew the oil so that it activates the saliva. Do this for at least 10 -15 minutes. The oil will turn white in your mouth as you do this. The oil pulls toxins and excess mucus out of the blood through the mucus membranes in the mouth.

Spit the oil out in the toilet. Again, Avoid **Swallowing the Oil**. After spitting, swish your mouth with a pinch of unrefined, mineral rich sea salt in warm purified water.

Immediately following the sea salt-water rinse, brush your teeth thoroughly. Use a tongue scraper to clean your tongue well, and then use a toothbrush to clean the roof of the mouth too.

Next, drink 2–3 glasses of purified (non-chlorinated and non- fluoridated) water.

The result will be a fresh, relaxed feeling. Gums will bleed less and teeth will get whiter.

If you do this on a continual basis, you may notice that dark, puffy circles under your eyes will start to disappear. You may even have more energy, a better memory, and a better night's sleep.

4
Raw and Living Foods

The key to health is a clean and nutrient-rich body. Raw, living foods are a great way to get there. Raw foods are foods that have not been heated over 105–118°F. In this form, the enzymes in the food retain much higher nutrient levels. We need enzymes for digestion and nutrient absorption. Live enzymes in foods ensure the food we eat is digested more efficiently and completely.

Raw and living foods are the best form of food for optimum health and wellness. These foods feed the body on a deep cellular level, without stressing the body as much as cooked food does. Cooked foods are essentially dead. They don't supply any live enzymes. So, your body has to work much harder by supplying more of its own enzyme store to digest your food. Working harder to supply the enzymes and then using them to digest the "enzyme-empty" food puts stress on the body. Simply eating foods that readily supply their own enzymes will greatly improve your digestion and overall health.

Raw and living foods make more nutrients available for the body during digestion. Raw foods are also highly alkalizing. The body's pH should ideally be around 7.2 or 7.3. Most people with chronic or acute diseases usually have overly acidic bodies. Eating foods that are highly alkalizing can help the body maintain a healthier pH, which leads to better health.

So what kinds of foods are in a raw and living food diet? A raw foods diet consists of unprocessed and uncooked (not heated over 105°F) fruits, vegetables, nuts, seeds, and grains. Fruit are slightly different from other foods. They are such a pure form of food that our digestive system processes them quickly compared to other foods. Therefore, it is best to eat fruit by itself and at least 15–30 minutes before eating other types of foods. Otherwise, digestion can stagnate.

Many people start eating raw foods to heal their bodies, or to just be healthier overall. However, some of my clients who adopted this diet on a 100% basis for a year or two said they were feeling weak and sick. If eating raw is taken to an extreme, it can create imbalances in the body and stress the thyroid, spleen, and pancreas.

Like anything else, balance is the key. Consuming a diet that varies the amount of raw food eaten, that is eaten in tune with the seasons, and that is eaten with your blood type in mind, can help to bring more balance to the body. Eating lighter raw foods (such as salads) in the warmer months and adding warmer foods (like soups and vegetable stews) in the colder months can be more supportive to certain people and to certain parts of the body.

For example, the thyroid can be supported better when cruciferous vegetables like broccoli and cauliflower are lightly steamed instead of eaten raw. This is because these foods (as well as a few others like yams, canola, and soy) contain natural chemicals called goitrogens that can interfere with thyroid hormone synthesis. Lightly steaming or cooking the vegetables will deactivate these chemicals. Adding foods like cooked whole-grain quinoa to the diet can work as a tonic for the spleen and pancreas.

A diet with a ratio of about 80% raw to 20% cooked food will work for most people for most of the year. Enjoy your raw foods, but remember to listen to your own body and create balance in your health, your diet, and your life. A good number of the recipes in this book are raw and living food recipes, which is a great place to start!

5
Fats and Oils

So what's the skinny on fats? Fat does not necessarily make us fat. In fact, the right kinds of fat can make us skinny, as well as support our overall health, and give us more energy. Fat is actually a critical component to our health.

When people tell me they need protein, I think what they probably need is the right fat in their diet. Their bodies are craving "good" fat. The advertising industry would have us believe that fat is bad or fattening. But in reality, good fat can be critical to our health and our weight management. Fat actually tells the body how to utilize proteins and carbohydrates. Fat in our food can make it taste more rich and satisfying. Many low-fat or fat-free products are filled with salt, sugar, chemical additives, and MSG to make up for the lack of flavorful fat.

Good fats are vital for good brain health. When I refer to "good" fats, I mean raw, unprocessed, organic fats in their natural form. Trans fats should always be avoided completely. Trans fats are hydrogenated fats that have been chemically changed into a non-natural or abnormal condition.

They will stay solid at room temperature and have unnaturally long shelf lives. These kinds of fats are unhealthy, even in tiny amounts.

Essential fatty acids are found in "good fats". These acids are called essential because they are not made by our body, and therefore must be obtained through the diet. Omega-6 and omega-3 are the specific essential fatty acids I'll address in this book.

We should all try to have a balance of omega-6 and omega-3 fats in our daily diet. Many doctors recommend a ratio of 3 to 1 (with omega-6 being the 3, and omega-3 being the 1). However, doctors at the Institute of Integrative Nutrition, affiliated with Columbia University, said the ratio really should be closer to 1 to 1. Most Americans get much more omega-6 than omega-3, so it may be important for you to become more aware of your fat intake. Really work on getting the proper amount of omega-3 essential fatty acids into your diet.

Omega-3 helps prevent many health problems because of their anti-inflammatory properties. This includes health problems such as heart disease, rheumatoid arthritis, macular degeneration, asthma, eczema, other immune dysfunctions, and cancer. Omega-3 also helps improve memory and can help improve mood. A deficiency in omega-3 may cause symptoms such as inflammation, water retention, and high blood pressure.

Luckily, there are many sources of good omega-3 fatty acids that, with just a little bit of extra effort, are easy to add to your diet. One example is high-quality nut and seed oils. I like raw, cold-pressed nut and seed oils. Pumpkin, walnut, flax, sesame, almond, hemp, and macadamia nut are some of my favorites. It is important to avoid heating most oils, as they can quickly become toxic. So, I only use them in recipes where they are not being heated. Or, if I do add them, it is after the food has been cooked and has cooled down.

The foods you make and eat will be more satisfying and delicious with the added health benefits of oils rich in omega-3. If you are worried about weight gain, these good fats can actually help with weight loss. The bad fats and other additives in processed foods are what cause ill health and weight problems.

Coconut oil is a type of nut fat. It is a saturated fat and a very chemically stable fat, meaning it can be heated without negative effects. It is also resistant to peroxidation and rancidity. Coconut oil is seen in most parts of the world as the super-food of fats. It is a unique saturated fat and a medium-chain fatty acid, meaning it doesn't need pancreatic enzymes or bile in order for the body to process it. Therefore, it is easily absorbed by the body. Coconut oil is also unique if you are a calorie counter. Coconut oil has 2.6% less calories per gram than other fats. It is also a great facilitator of energy.

Coconut oil nourishes the body, and the medium-chained fatty acids provide a good source of energy. Coconut oil is also highly effective as an antioxidant. Additionally, the unique lauric acid naturally occurring in coconut oil is a natural and powerful immune system booster.[6]

Coconut oil is a unique, healthy fat. It is a safe alternative oil for any cooking recipe. The Natural Gourmet Institute for Food and Health always uses coconut oil whenever cooking with heat. I learned this when I was there taking my health-supportive cooking class. Very few oils handle heat well, but certain coconut oils handle high heat very well. Read labels and make certain you are purchasing the type that is meant to handle whichever cooking method you require. Some that are more refined will say whether they are meant for cooking with high heat.

For years, coconut oil had a bad rap. It was widely believed that coconut oil was bad for health because it raised cholesterol. In actuality, it provides "good" cholesterol (HDL).

A meta-analysis published in the *American Journal of Clinical Nutrition*, March 2010, found that "dietary saturated fats aren't associated with heart diseases and stroke." The researchers examined data from almost 350,000 people, who were followed for up to 23 years. The study showed no relationship between saturated fat intake and the risk of cardiovascular diseases and stroke.[7]

A March, 2008 article published in the *American Journal of Clinical Nutrition* presented a study of 49 overweight women and men. They were put on a calorie-restrictive diet using either MCT fat (pure coconut oil is MCT) or olive oil as the type of fat in the diet. Both groups lost weight, but the group that consumed MCT fat lost an average of seven pounds. The group using olive oil only lost an average of three pounds. In weight loss studies, the people eating MCT fats reported feeling more satisfied and having more energy after eating. Increased postprandial thermogenesis and energy expenditure have been observed in both lean and obese subjects.[8]

These results are in line with other similar studies showing a reduction in weight and body fat in overweight participants who consumed MCT oil as part of their diet. Many participants involved in some of the weight-loss studies using coconut or MCT oil also reported higher satiety and more stable energy levels, which can facilitate weight loss. This is because the unique structure of MCT fats in coconut oil makes them easier to burn and harder to store in adipose tissues, compared to the LCFAs found in most other fats, including olive oil.[9]

Pure coconut oil is known as a functional food and has many benefits in addition to its nutritional value. Here are some examples:

- Promoting your heart health
- Supporting your immune system health
- Supporting a healthy metabolism
- Providing you with an immediate energy source
- Helping to keep your skin healthy and looking youthful
- Supporting the proper functioning of your thyroid gland

Coconut oil appears to be unique in its ability to help with brain function. Recently, I read about how Dr. Mary T. Newport cured her husband of Alzheimer's disease. She began adding coconut oil to his diet, and asserted this to be one of the main components of his cure. So, what is Alzheimer's disease, and why would coconut oil help?

Alzheimer's disease "appears to be a type of diabetes of the brain, and it's a process that starts happening at least 10 or 20 years before you start having symptoms. It's also very similar to type 1 or type 2 diabetes in that you develop a problem with insulin. In this case, insulin problems prevent brain cells from accepting glucose, their primary fuel. Without it, they eventually die. But there is an alternative fuel: ketones, which cells easily accept. Ketones metabolize in the liver after you eat medium-chain triglycerides, like those found in coconut oil."[10]

Many of my recipes call for coconut oil. Make sure you purchase organic, extra-virgin, pure coconut oil. You do not want to purchase or confuse pure coconut oil with a hydrogenated or trans fat variety.

Canola Oil

Canola is a brand name. It is a plant in Canada developed from the rapeseed plant, which is a member of the mustard family. It is used in many products and foods, because it is apparently low in saturated fats and has a high proportion of monounsaturated fats. I have seen advertisements saying it is all right to use when cooking with heat. Never heat oil (any oil) over its smoking point. The smoke produced can be toxic. Many foods prepared at restaurants, stores, and bakeries have canola oil as an ingredient.

The erucic acid levels in rapeseed oil are said to be toxic. Rapeseed oil contains about 30–60% erucic acid. Canola oil has been developed to contain less than 2% erucic acid.[11] Canola oil is fairly new. It hasn't been around long enough to have its long term and short term effects on humans and animals studied and completely understood. Canola oil has been the subject of much controversy. I personally never use nor recommend canola oil.

Olive Oil

Olive oil is a wonderful and unique ingredient. It is an omega-9 oil, a monounsaturated fat, a long-chained fatty acid, and the only vegetable oil that can be pressed and used in its pure form. The key ingredient found in olive oil is oleic acid. Some studies have shown oleic acid to aid in cancer protection and prevention.

Olive oil is a good fat, and is a staple in a healthy Mediterranean diet. However, olive oil can become rancid if heated or stored improperly. It needs to be kept cool (or refrigerated) and away from light. In fact, all nut, seed, and vegetable oils should be kept refrigerated and away from light.

Olive oil should be used only with non-cooking recipes and food preparation, unless it says on the label that it is meant to handle high heat. More refined varieties of olive oils can handle certain high temperatures. When olive oil (or any oil, for that matter) is heated beyond what is known as the smoke point, the oil can become toxic.

George Mateljan (a biologist, businessman, and nutritionist best known for his book *The World's Healthiest Foods*) told Jen Weigel, an independent writer for *Chicago Now,* that "olive oil should be heated below 250°F. Otherwise, toxic fumes can be created from oil that is overheated. People are inhaling this smoke every day when they think it's being healthy, but in reality, the smoke from heated olive oil is full of toxins."[12]

Ms. Weigel followed up with George about olive oil. She said, "I emailed George to ask him about this, as well as whether or not you can bake with olive oil without the toxic smoke, since that was also a concern to many. He said that yes indeed, he does not recommend heating olive oil above 200–250°F. He says that you can bake with olive oil up to 350°F degrees, and it will not smoke because the molecules are surrounded by moisture and dough." When some people questioned Weigel's article, she said,

> Dr. Oz did his food "Hall of Shame" episode, and suddenly, I was validated. He listed many foods to avoid in order to be your best self and stay healthy. In this video clip from Oprah.com, he mentions that you should *not* cook healthy oils, because "when you have healthy oils, and you cook with them, you damage them.... Healthy oils would be olive oil, sesame oil, canola oil, or flaxseed oil." ...While olive oil can and should be a healthy part of your diet, what most people do not appreciate is that olive oil should not be used to cook with.

If you are using olive oil for non-cooked recipes, choose organic, extra-virgin olive oil, which is from the first press of the olive. Extra-virgin olive oil has more Vitamin E in it than other types of olive oil. Olive oil "is a monounsaturated fat, and it contains major health benefits because of its vitamin E and

A, chlorophyll, magnesium, squalene and a host of other cardio-protective nutrients. It has also been shown to reduce some cancers, as well as rheumatoid arthritis."[13]

Hemp Oil

Hemp oil contains significant amounts of omega-3s and omega-6s. Hemp oil also contains significant amounts of Vitamin E, which is important for the thyroid gland. One easy thing you can do for your diet is to freshly grind hemp or flax seeds and add them to recipes for an extra boost of omega oils, as well as protein and fiber.

Flax Seeds

Flax seeds are one of the best sources of omega-3 essential fatty acids. Flax seeds are rich with alpha-linolenic acid, fiber, and lignans. Lignans are phytoestrogens or plant compounds that have an estrogen-like effect with antioxidant properties. These lignans can help stabilize hormone levels and reduce pre-menstrual syndrome and menopause symptoms. They can also potentially help reduce the risk of developing prostate or breast cancer. The alpha-linolenic acid is anti-inflammatory. It promotes the lowering of the C-reactive protein in the blood, which is a biomarker of inflammation. Freshly grind flax seeds when using them to get the full benefit of the oil. Do not buy flax seeds that are already ground. Store flax seeds in a dry, waterproof container. Always store ground seeds in the refrigerator.

Chia Seeds

Chia seeds are an ancient seed cultivated for thousands of years in Mexico. The word "chia" means strength. Unlike flax seeds and hemp seeds, chia seeds do not have to be ground up in order for the body to utilize the nutrients and oils, making them much easier for the body to use. Chia seeds have more omega-3 fatty acids than Atlantic salmon, but unlike the salmon, chia seeds are also are about 10% omega-6 oil, so they are a more ideal balance of omega fats. Chia seeds are 3 omega-3s to 1 omega-6. Along with the rich omega oils, chia seeds also have four times more calcium than milk (1 ounce of chia has 179 mg. calcium, and 1 ounce of whole milk has 36 mg. calcium), more antioxidants than fresh blueberries, and more protein, calcium, and fiber than flax seeds. Chia seeds are one of the best nutrient-dense superfoods around.

Chia seeds, ground flax seeds, or ground hemp seeds can provide omega-3s. You can also buy omega-3 flax seed oil at the grocery store. Omega-6 essential fatty acids need to be balanced with omega-3 essential fatty acids. An excess of omega-6 can cause water retention, raised blood pressure, and increased blood clotting.

Choose organic, whole-food, cold-pressed, non-processed vegetarian "good" fats and enjoy your food. Don't feel guilty about adding healthy fat to recipes. Your body and your brain will be glad you did!

6
Sugar and Sweeteners

We find sugar everywhere, presented in the most beautiful, innocent ways supported by societal norms. Sugar is one of the most harmful ingredients in our diet. Sugar is found in almost all processed and fast foods. Sugar can feed cancer and other diseases. Sugar intake also can lead to hypoglycemia, cardiovascular disease, weight gain, diabetes, kidney disease, high blood pressure, tooth decay, systemic infections, memory disorders, allergies, and hormonal imbalances.

Refined sugars, high-fructose corn syrup, and fructose are all hard on the body and the digestive system. Simple carbs, like refined sugar and high-fructose corn syrup (excepting fruit sugar), are more easily converted into glucose because their molecular structure breaks down faster in the stomach and small intestine. Therefore, these carbs raise glucose levels in the bloodstream quite rapidly (in less than 30 minutes). This quick rise in blood sugar can put a good deal of stress on the pancreas, which will try to regulate the sudden spike in blood sugar by producing insulin to control it.

White, refined carbohydrates, sugar, and high-fructose corn syrup are read by the body as empty simple sugars. The empty sugar will also make the body pull nutrients from the body in order to process it. Sugar can be hiding in many foods, so be sure to read each list of ingredients carefully.

Here are a few types of sweeteners that are alternatives to refined sugar and high-fructose corn syrup:

Stevia is a sweet plant from South America. Japanese food manufacturers developed this alternative sweetener from the stevia plant in the 1970s for use in their products. The Japanese have done extensive research on stevia and found it to be safe. The less-refined varieties of stevia are the best in terms of health benefits. Stevia has no calories and low glycemic properties. This sweetener is probably one of the best choices for diabetics to use. I like the liquid variety best. I have found that the powdered form of stevia has a somewhat bitter aftertaste.

Check the stevia packaging carefully to see what ingredients are in it. I found one that had grapefruit seed extract used as a preservative. A client of mine was using it and, because of his medication, this grapefruit ingredient could have killed him.

Instead of powdered stevia, I prefer to use xylitol powder; if I need to use a packet of powdered sweetener.

Xylitol is a sugar alcohol found in fruits and vegetables. It is made from birch tree bark and other hard wood trees. Finland used this sugar during World War II when they had a sugar shortage. Germany, Switzerland, Japan, and the Soviet Union were using xylitol by the 1960s extensively. It was their preferred sweetener for diabetics.

Many studies have been done on xylitol. It has been shown to help prevent cavities, repair dental enamel, regulate blood sugar for those with Type 2 diabetes, strengthen bones, decrease age-related bone loss, inhibit systemic yeast problems, inhibit the growth of bacteria that cause middle-ear infections in children, and inhibit the growth of strep. Xylitol has fewer calories and 75% fewer carbohydrates than sugar. Studies have shown that ingesting xylitol can alkalize your body, reduce sugar cravings, and reduce insulin levels. It was approved by the FDA in 1963.

(Note: **Xylitol is toxic to pets.**)

> **Artificial Sweeteners: Chemically derived sweeteners can have a harmful effect on health.**

Aspartame is the technical name for what makes up the artificial sweeteners NutraSweet, Equal, Spoonful, and Equal-Measure. It is composed of three chemicals: aspartic acid, phenylalanine, and methanol.

Aspartame can cause many problems, including neurological ones. Here's an example:

When the temperature of aspartame exceeds 86°F, the wood alcohol in aspartame converts to formaldehyde and then to formic acid, which in turn causes metabolic acidosis. The methanol toxicity mimics multiple sclerosis; thus, people may be misdiagnosed with having multiple sclerosis. Multiple sclerosis does not lead to death whereas methanol toxicity does.[14]

According to a report from the National Institutes of Health:

Methanol is extremely poisonous. As little as two tablespoons can be deadly to a child. About 2 to 8 ounces can be deadly for an adult. Blindness is common and often permanent despite medical care. How well the person recovers depends on how much poison is swallowed and how soon treatment is received.[15]

In a 2003 memo to the FDA, on the subject of recalling aspartame as a neurotoxic drug, Mark Gold of the Aspartame Toxicity Information Center reported:

Both the U.S. Air Force's magazine *Flying Safety* and the U.S. Navy's magazine *Navy Physiology* published articles warning about the many dangers of aspartame including the cumulative deleterious effects of methanol and the greater likelihood of birth defects. The articles note the ingestion of aspartame may make pilots more susceptible to seizures and vertigo (US Air Force, 1992). Countless other toxicity effects have been reported to the FDA (DHHS, 1995), other independent organizations (Mission Possible, 1996; Stoddard, 1995), and independent scientists (e.g., 80 cases of seizures were reported to Dr. Richard Wurtman, Food (1986)).[16]

Gold continues in his memo:
Examples of aspartame toxicity reactions can be found on the Aspartame (NutraSweet) Toxicity Info Center web page:
http://www.tiac.net/users/mgold/aspartame/

Frequently, aspartame toxicity is misdiagnosed as a specific disease. This hasn't been reported in the scientific literature, yet it has been reported countless times to independent organizations and scientists. In other cases, it has been reported that chronic aspartame ingestion has triggered or worsened certain chronic illnesses. Nearly 100% of the time, the patient and physician assume these worsening conditions are simply a normal progression of the illness. Sometimes that may be true, but many times it is chronic aspartame poisoning.

According to researchers and physicians studying the adverse effects of aspartame, the following list contains a selection of chronic illnesses that may be caused or worsened by the chronic, long-term ingestion of aspartame:

- Brain tumors
- Multiple sclerosis
- Epilepsy
- Chronic fatigue syndrome
- Parkinson's disease
- Alzheimer's
- Mental retardation
- Lymphoma
- Birth defects
- Fibromyalgia
- Diabetes
- Arthritis (including Rheumatoid)
- Chemical sensitivities
- Attention Deficit Disorder

Note: In some cases such as MS, the severe symptoms mimic the illness or exacerbate the illness but do not cause the disease.[17]

Note that this is an incomplete list. Clearly, ingestion of a slow poison is not beneficial to anyone who has a chronic illness.

From my research, I conclude that avoiding artificial sweeteners in any amount would be wise and prudent. Instead, stick with real, whole, unrefined, or unprocessed sugars as much as possible. Read ingredient labels carefully, and check for any sugar or sugar substitute.

Sadly, even doing that isn't always reliable. The Federal Drug Administration (FDA) allows artificial sweeteners to be added to such foods as dairy products without stating the name of the artificial sweetener on the label if it is added under a certain percentage. This lets manufacturers claim the product has fewer calories and less sugar than similar products. This should not be allowed! *All ingredients should be listed on the ingredients label. Period.*

It's a trick to make consumers think that fewer calories, less sugar, or "low fat" is healthier when in actuality, adding harmful ingredients is worse than full fat or natural calories in food. I say, demand full disclosure of what's in our food. If we don't *demand* it, then it won't happen. We consumers should be able to know what's in our food supply. Let our voices be heard. That is the only way lawmakers know we even care.

7
Salt

When I ask people if they use salt, they frequently tell me, "No, I eat a low-salt diet for health reasons." In fact, it is not salt that is bad for us, it is the *type* of salt we eat. The word "electrolyte" is a chemical term for salt. We need electrolytes to be healthy. As Dr. David Brownstein says, "Without salt, life itself would not be possible.[18] The misconception about salt stems from the fact that conventional medical doctors make no differentiation between white, refined salt and unrefined, mineral-rich sea salt.

Unrefined sea salt is important for life because it: promotes the proper balance for the endocrine, adrenal, and thyroid gland to function properly; supports healthy blood pressure; detoxifies the body; and, along with water, is necessary for the optimal functioning of the immune system, hormonal system, and cardiovascular health.[19] When we sweat, our body can lose many minerals, and these minerals need to be replenished. Unrefined whole sea salt contains these minerals. Sea salt can also help balance the body by alkalizing it. Maintaining a slightly alkaline pH is important to our health.

The white refined table salt most of us grew up using lacks numerous minerals that are present in whole, natural sea salt. Refined table salt is 98 percent sodium chloride with added bicarbonates, chemicals, sugar, and preservatives. Iodine, the main nutrient that supports our thyroid gland, is added to many refined salts, but in insufficient quantities "to prevent thyroid illnesses or to provide for the body's iodine needs."[20] Given that iodine dissipates after being exposed to oxygen, table salt could never be a reliable source of iodine anyway.

Many food sources today lack vital minerals and nutrients. Soils are depleted, and refining and processing take out many or all of the nutrients in foods. Salt cravings are actually a signal you may be depleted in nutrients, minerals, and electrolytes. Salt cravings can also be a signal that your thyroid and adrenal glands need minerals. If you have been craving salt or have been under a good deal of stress, have your thyroid checked to make sure you are getting enough iodine in your diet. We don't have many food sources for iodine, and it can be extremely important to our health.

Dr. Brownstein says low-salt diets "promote toxicity" and have:

> . . .adverse effects on numerous metabolic markers, including promoting elevated insulin levels and insulin resistance. Low-salt diets have been associated with elevating normal

cholesterol and LDL cholesterol levels, which in turn, have been associated with cardiovascular disease. Finally, low-salt diets will lead to mineral deficiencies and the development of chronic disease.[21]

In 1994, The *British Medical Journal* published a study conducted in the Netherlands. The study examined 100 men and women between the ages of 55 and 75 who had mild to moderate hypertension. When common, refined table salt was replaced with mineral salt high in magnesium and potassium, the study showed a reduction in blood pressure equivalent to that produced by drugs which lower blood pressure.[22]

There are various types of sea salt with different mineral contents. Try a few different ones and see which you like the best. Celtic sea salt is supposed to be high in minerals, and I like to use Bolivian Rose salt as well. Try to buy a solar-dried salt or a mined salt. Mined salt may be cleaner and more nutrient-dense because it was formed when oceans were less polluted, and during a more nutrient-dense time.

8
Nutrients, Additives, and Preservatives

Iodine is one of the most important nutrients to support our health. Iodine is an essential nutrient that supports the thyroid, our "master gland" which is central to all of our body's major functions. The thyroid, located in the bottom middle of the front of our neck, influences our metabolism, weight, digestion, energy, body temperature, skin, hair, sleep, mental acuity, nervous system, sexual organs, and hormonal system. In fact, it would be very difficult to find a system that is not influenced by the thyroid. Because of the thyroid's widespread effects, its malfunction can significantly affect a person's life and pose a detriment to long-term health.

It is difficult to have a healthy thyroid without iodine. So, what foods contain iodine? That is a good question. Because our soil is pretty much depleted of this nutrient, few foods actually contain iodine. Chlorine and fluoride in the water can also cause iodine deficiency. Please try to keep those chemicals out of your water, shower, and food.

Until 1980, bakeries added iodine to bread. After 1980, they switched to adding potassium bromate. What does this mean? We have a certain amount of space for iodine in our thyroid. Our body can store about three months' worth of iodine in the cells. When we ingest potassium bromate, also called bromide, it acts like iodine and takes up the space in the thyroid reserved for iodine. This prevents the body from absorbing the iodine it needs. The chlorine and fluoride that almost all municipal water companies in the United States put in water act the same way. These chemicals can all contribute to iodine deficiency.

Iodine is added to table salt. However, when it is exposed to oxygen, the iodine dissipates, so table salt is not really a reliable source of iodine. Also, table salt is actually refined sodium with added sugar, bicarbonates, chemicals, and preservatives. The minerals are removed, and the body reads this table salt as toxic chemicals.

Because I know how important iodine is for our health, I created my own unrefined, natural iodine-containing sea salt seasoning for me and my family. It is now available on my website. This is a sea salt seasoning that you use in place of regular table salt when seasoning your food. Whole, organic, raw, mineral-rich and nutrient-dense non-refined sea salt seasoning mixture. This unprocessed food has an abundance of healthful nutrients, including rich iodine, which supports the thyroid gland, our master gland.

If you are concerned about iodine or your thyroid, then I recommend reading Dr. David Brownstein's book *Overcoming Thyroid Disorders*. Weight problems can be a direct result of a thyroid problem, and they are misdiagnosed regularly. I also believe the synthetic types of thyroid supplement can be harmful, so read his book and look at his recommendations. It is excellent and very short.

Watch Out For Sulfites

Sulfites are preservatives added to many foods, drinks, and medicines. In fact, they have been used for centuries as a preservative, because they preserve the color and flavor by inhibiting the growth of bacteria. Symptoms of sulfite allergy include weight gain, or the inability to lose weight, and respiratory types of problems. Many people who have been struggling with their weight find that, after cutting out sulfites, they can lose weight much more easily and then keep it off.

The most reliable way to test for a sulfite allergy is to go on a totally non-sulfite diet for several weeks. Because sulfites are hidden in many foods, you may have to eat nothing but whole, organic, non-sulfite or sulfate-agent-containing foods for three weeks. (Sulfite agents take the form of sodium sulfite, sodium bisulfite, sodium metabisulfite, metabisulfite, potassium bisulfate, and potassium metabisulfites.) If all of your symptoms disappear, then you may be allergic to sulfites or other additives in the foods you cut out of your diet. Some doctors may want to give you a pill containing sulfites to see if the symptoms reoccur, just to confirm the allergy. This should only be done under close supervision.

If you are allergic to sulfites, then you can simply regulate your diet accordingly, to avoid sulfites. The USDA requires any food containing 10ppm or more of sulfites to be labeled. But, since the labels on many foods change periodically, read the labels each time you buy processed food products. Look out for sulfite, sodium bisulfite, sodium metabisulfite, potassium bisulfite, and potassium metabisulfite on ingredient labels.

Foods that commonly add sulfites to their ingredients are soups, canned vegetables, dried fruits, bakery items, pickles, potato chips, condiments, trail mixes, shrimp, and guacamole. The FDA passed a law in 1986 banning the use of sulfites on raw fruits and vegetables.

Vitamin C, quercetin, and bromelain are vitamins commonly used to aid in the treatment of sulfite allergies. Vitamin C and quercetin are immune system boosters. Bromelain will help your body use quercetin. Quercetin is also known for its ability to block the release of histamines, so it helps with any allergy symptoms.

You may find you feel much better after you cut sulfites out of your diet. Removing the chemicals and preservatives out of the food you eat is a huge step toward getting healthier and thinner. Many of us grew up thinking additives are "normal" to ingest. But, in my opinion, God did not make our bodies to assimilate chemicals and preservatives. Did God make a little baby and then say, "Please give this baby chemicals and preservatives for nourishment"? Whole, real food that is grown, harvested, and stored in a safe and healthy way is what I believe we are meant to have as nourishment for our body.

9
Slimming Secrets

We all want to be in the best physical shape we can be, whether it's for wearing a swimsuit in summer or a party outfit for the winter holidays. Here is a wonderfully easy way to slim down and create the energy and vitality you want for those activities!

First of all, this weight loss slimming plan includes vegetables in their natural, raw state. A raw, uncooked vegetable, thoroughly chewed and swallowed, then assimilated, will create a set of carbozyme slimming actions!

Eat the leaves of vegetables for fast weight loss, including spinach, chard, beet greens, turnip greens, Chinese cabbage, mustard greens, Brussels sprouts, cabbage, and kale. These carbozymes will burn up unwanted fat cells quickly. Enzymes in raw foods, such as fruits, vegetables, seeds, and nuts act by stabilizing the metabolism, which increases control of the secretory processes. This creates an inhibitory effect on appetite and maintains a normal desire for food. Raw food enzymes soothe the hunger urge and control the gastric secretions, resulting in a decreased desire to overeat.

Second, eat a raw vegetable (carrot, radish, bell pepper, or celery) about 10–15 minutes before a meal. Eat and chew it thoroughly. The carbozymes in the raw vegetables will promote the formation of red blood cells, plus stimulate respiration and nitrogen metabolism of the cell tissues. This creates better metabolism of protein, normalized blood pressure, corrected pancreatic function, and improved circulation. This all adds up to better health while slimming down. Raw vegetables offer carbozymes that alert the metabolism to help cleanse the heavy, weighty molecules that cling to the adipose cell tissues. With this catalyst action, the adipose cells are cleansed of the stored-up fats and calories.

Those are the two main things to do. But, as you do those, try to eat a rainbow of food colors daily. The antioxidants are in the color pigment! Try to eat colorful, fresh, seasonal foods year round.

Third, when you eat, take your time. Sit down. Really enjoy and chew your food well. Enzymes need time to help raise your blood sugar. Try replacing a coffee break with a raw juice or green smoothie break. If hungry, try a glass of tomato juice or munch on celery, carrots, radishes or pickles. These offer enzymes to help control appetite. Think and concentrate on your food.

Fourth, try to have a protein at every meal. Enzymes, for the metabolic process to keep weight off and control your appetite, use protein. I bet you didn't know leafy greens are a great source of protein. Spinach is 45% protein.

In conclusion, slim down by eating delicious, raw, or lightly steamed vegetables, and have the vitality and radiant health you always wanted!

10
Vegetarianism and Health

Plant-based foods can be very healing to the body. Plant-based foods in their natural form can help alkalize the body, as well as nourish the body in a healthy way. Most of the recipes I have in my books are vegetarian. I'm a vegetarian, and I've found it helps my health immensely. I'm not saying everyone should be a vegetarian, but the more plant-based foods you add to your diet, the healthier you become.

According to the ADA[23], vegetarians are at lower risk for developing:

- Heart disease.
- Colorectal, ovarian, and breast cancers.
- Diabetes.
- Obesity.
- Hypertension (high blood pressure).[24]

Dr. Caldwell B. Esselstyn, Jr., former president of the medical staff at the Cleveland Clinic, writes that you can reverse heart disease with no drugs and only a plant-based diet, based on the groundbreaking results of his 20-year nutritional study. Backed up by solid scientific evidence, he argues that we can end the heart disease epidemic by changing what we eat. Dr. Esselstyn recommends a plant-based, oil-free diet that he says can prevent heart disease, stop its progress, and even reverse its effects.[25]

The late Walter Kempner, MD, founded the Rice Diet. He believed that a diet of rice, fruit, and vegetables did miraculous things for people, and helped them to gain back their health. He treated hundreds of people at Duke University, where he prescribed a diet of rice, vegetables and fruit that reversed hypertension, diabetic eye changes, heart failure, kidney failure, and obesity.[26]

Working from a scientific basis, Dr. T. Colin Campbell, PhD, professor emeritus at Cornell University and co-author of *The China Study*, the most comprehensive human nutrition study to date, advocates a plant-based diet for optimum health. I was fortunate to be part of Dr. Campbell's class at Cornell University, where he told us:

Plant-based eating is a superior way of eating. Benefits of eating this way: you will live longer; look and feel younger; have more energy; lose weight; lower your blood cholesterol; prevent and even reverse heart disease; lower your risk of prostate, breast, and other cancers; preserve your eyesight in your later years; prevent and treat diabetes; avoid surgery; vastly decrease your need for pharmaceutical drugs; keep your bones strong; avoid impotence; avoid stroke; prevent kidney stones; keep your baby from getting type II diabetes; alleviate constipation; lower your blood pressure; avoid Alzheimer's; beat arthritis, and more.

Dr. Campbell discussed the studies he had done on the diseases that arise in populations when meat protein is introduced into the diet. He continued:

My early research gave me the understanding that animal protein, when tested experimentally, was substantially different from plant protein in its ability to promote tumor development. It turned out that animal protein had its effect by operating through a constellation of integrative mechanisms. The division between animal and plant foods was a signpost of a division of the kinds of foods having an effect on cancer.[27]

In Dr. Campbell's class on plant-based nutrition, I learned of many studies that prove it is possible to be healthy or overcome illness on a plant-based diet. Recently, one such study conducted by a team of American and Japanese researchers showed that people who have diabetes can vastly improve their health by eating an entirely plant-based diet.[28] More than 100 million people today have diabetes or pre-diabetes. The study's findings concur with my experience. During my work with people who have diabetes, I have found that they show remarkable improvement in their health and well-being from consuming a plant-based and almost completely raw food diet.

For that study, the researchers also undertook a new meta-analysis in which they compared six significant prior research studies. The researchers found that a plant-based diet significantly improved blood sugar control in type 2 diabetes and specifically in a key indicator of blood sugar control called hemoglobin A1c. The participants' results improved as much as 1.2 points, which was greater than the effect of typical oral diabetes medicines.

The study also combined the results of all of the available studies. It indicated that the benefits of excluding dairy products (including cheese), eggs, and meat from the diet was as much as 0.7 points in some studies, and averaging 0.4 points overall. The participants in most of these studies were not required to reduce their calorie or carbohydrate consumption.[29]

Everyone needs to find the diet that works best for them, and find balance in their life. I also know that the quality of the food we eat is vital. From my studies, I believe an organic, plant-based diet can benefit your health immensely, and even heal your body.

11
Bed Time

Night time can be a time when you really nurture yourself. Treat yourself like you are the special person you are. I recommend unwinding at the end of the day. It helps us relax and therefore sleep more peacefully. At the end of the day, I recommend putting on some calming lights, maybe playing some nice instrumental music, and writing down your to-do list for tomorrow to get it off your mind and out of your brain. Relax.

While you are doing this, you can fill a bathtub with warm water, adding two cups of Epsom salts and ½ cup of baking soda. The salt sulfates will absorb into the skin and help your body create glutathione, which is a detoxifying molecule. You can add a few drops of lavender or some relaxing essential oil right before you step in to the bath. If you add it too soon, it will dissipate before you get in.

Then, take this warm, comforting, relaxing, cleansing bath about half an hour before bed. Avoid any computer or cell phone work for an hour before bed. The blue LED lights in electronics can affect the melatonin levels in your body and prevent you from getting a restful and healing night's sleep. If you can, put them outside your bedroom, so their electromagnetic fields won't disturb your body's energy.

If you have allergies, or have problems sleeping due to difficulty breathing, I recommend and personally use an air decontamination machine. It makes the oxygen in the air more bio available, while also continually eliminating viruses, mold, bacteria, and fungus on soft surfaces (bedding, pet beds, carpet, and clothing) and hard surfaces as well. This technology is an advanced solution for eliminating odors, decontaminating surfaces and purifying the air in your home, office, or RV. It is a totally green technology. For more information: Go to "my products" in "my store" at www.organichealthylifestyle.com. There are portable systems and an in-duct system. (This technology has been approved by the FDA for medical facilities.)

After your relaxing bath, go to bed for a healing and restful night's sleep.

12
Basic Daily Menu Flow

Meals should be vegetarian and mostly whole, raw food, all organic, GMO-free, and as gluten-free as possible.

Note: First thing in morning, have a large glass of water.

Breakfast
- <u>One</u> of the following:
    - salad
    - soup
    - green smoothie
    - green vegetable juice

Wait 1½ hours after breakfast and drink ¼ your body weight (in pounds) in ounces of pure water.

Snacks
- 1 pint of green vegetable juice and, if necessary, some raw nuts or seeds

Wait 30 minutes after the snack and drink four ounces of rejuvelac.

Lunch
- Salad or soup
- Entrée
- Raw nut pâté or hummus
  - For chips, use raw vegetables or whole grain, gluten-free crackers.

Wait 1½ hours after lunch and drink at least ¼ your weight in pure water in ounces. Wait 30 minutes more and drink four ounces rejuvelac.

Dinner
- Salad & soup

13
Recipes

Recipes 1:
Drinks

Rejuvelac

Rejuvelac is a probiotic drink made with fermented seeds or grains. Probiotic means "for life". Most of the immune system is made up of probiotics. We need to replenish the probiotics in our body on a regular, ongoing basis. This drink is just as easy to make as it is easy to drink. An adult would typically drink eight, four-ounce servings per day (32 ounces total).

Notes:
You can purchase sprouted quinoa, or you can soak un-sprouted quinoa overnight in non-chlorinated water to remove the phytic acid. You do *not* need to soak the quinoa seeds *if they are already sprouted.*

Ingredients and equipment:
1 cup organic, non-GMO (genetically modified) quinoa, sprouted.
1 gallon high-quality water
Optional: ½ tsp. organic whey, or ¼ tsp. organic apple cider vinegar
1-gallon glass container
1 small piece of cheesecloth
1 large rubber band
1 large spoon

Directions:

1. Soak quinoa (if not already sprouted) in non-chlorinated water over night for 12–18 hours. Add ½ tsp. whey protein (or a ¼ tsp. of organic apple cider vinegar) to the water to better remove the phytic acid.

2. After soaking the quinoa, rinse the quinoa in a fine mesh colander (sieve) with running water.

3. Put the rinsed grain in the gallon jar.

4. Fill the jar up with the non-chlorinated pure water. If using purified water that is devoid of minerals, add ¼ tsp. whole unrefined mineral rich sea salt to the water. (Electrolyte is a fancy term for salt. Water needs these minerals for our body to optimally absorb it.)

5. Cover the jar top with the cheesecloth.

6. Please the rubber band around the top of the jar to hold the cheesecloth in place.

7. Stir the mixture once a day with the spoon and replace the cheesecloth.

8. The rejuvelac will ferment for about 2 days.

9. After 2 days, pour the mixture out, using a sieve or colander. Save the liquid. The liquid is the rejuvelac. This is the liquid probiotic you will drink.

10. You can cook this quinoa immediately and eat it as a meal or side dish.

11. The rejuvelac will last about a week in the refrigerator. If you are drinking 32 ounces a day, this recipe will last you four days.

Basic Green Juice Drink

Notes:
- This drink requires a juicer.
- If you are an O blood type, you may want to add a couple tablespoons of the pulp back into the drink after juicing. I also recommend adding a teaspoon of cold pressed flax oil or hemp seed oil to the juice before drinking.

Ingredients:
5 stalks celery
1 cucumber
2 leaves of kale
½ lemon with skin
1 pinch sea salt

Directions:
1. Juice all vegetables.
2. Add the pinch of sea salt to the drink before drinking.
3. Drink within 20 minutes.

Vegetable Juice Drink

Notes:

- This drink requires a juicer.
- If you are an O blood type, you may want to add a couple of tablespoons of the pulp back into the drink after juicing. I also recommend adding a teaspoon of cold pressed flax or hemp seed oil to the juice before drinking.

Ingredients:

4 stalks celery
½ cucumber
4 large leaves of kale or romaine lettuce
3 carrots
1 pinch of sea salt

Directions:

1. Juice all vegetables.
2. Add the pinch of sea salt to the drink before drinking.
3. Drink within 20 minutes.

Green Smoothie

Ingredients:
½ or 1 avocado (peeled, pitted, and diced)
1 cup baby kale, baby spinach, or romaine lettuce (chopped)
½ cucumber (chopped into chunks)
½ cup sprouts (ex. broccoli, radish, pea)
½ dropper plain liquid Stevia
1½ cups purified or spring water
½ tsp. unrefined, whole sea salt

Directions:
1. Blend all ingredients in a blender until smooth.
2. Drink within 20 minutes.

Variation:
Add 1 tablespoon maca root. Maca root is excellent for boosting libido and helping the body deal with stress.

Recipes 2:
Salad Dressings

Salads are a great choice for your menu and healthy eating plan. But store-bought salad dressings can be high in added sugar, and many of them contain canola oil. Avoid dressings with added sugar, high-fructose corn syrup, agave, or canola oil.

Sometimes I simply squeeze the juice of a lemon or lime on my salad to make a delicious, easy, and healthy salad dressing.

Adding sliced avocado, sliced mushrooms, tomatoes, sprouted seeds and nuts, or fresh micro-greens or sprouts can make leafy greens more interesting and much healthier. Keep it vegan if you want to lose weight faster or more effectively.

The following easy, delicious salad dressing recipes require a blender, will make two servings, and will keep for two days if refrigerated. Serve them over greens or chopped vegetables.

Good nutritious greens are: green lettuce, baby spinach, baby kale, watercress, and red leaf lettuce. Put a variety of these greens together for a symphony of flavor and a delicious, nourishing meal or side salad. Avoid iceberg lettuce, as it has very little nutritional value.

Cucumber Dressing

This was one of Larry Hagman's favorite recipes I made for him.

Ingredients:
1 cucumber (chopped into chunks with skin)
1 avocado (peeled, pitted, and diced)
1 tsp. unpasteurized apple cider vinegar or rice vinegar
¼ tsp. unrefined sea salt

Directions:
1. Blend all ingredients in a blender until smooth.
2. Store in the refrigerator in a glass jar with a tight lid.

Note:
Add a little bit of water to this if it's too thick.

Sweet Pepper Dressing

Ingredients:

1 red or yellow bell pepper (stem and seeds removed, chopped into chunks)
1 tomato (stem removed, chopped into chunks)
½ cup cold-pressed, unrefined flax or hemp seed oil
½ cup cilantro (fresh)
¼ tsp. unrefined sea salt

Directions:

1. Blend all ingredients in a blender until smooth.
2. Store in the refrigerator in a glass jar with a tight lid.

Creamy Italian Dressing

This is a very rich salad dressing, so just use it lightly for your salad.

Notes: Start this dressing recipe the day *before* you want to use it, because it is best to soak the nuts overnight. The soaking removes the phytic acid if you are using raw nuts.

Ingredients:

⅓ cup raw Brazil nuts (Soak in pure water overnight, then pour off the soaking water.)
¾ or 1 small cucumber (chopped with skin)
⅓ cup olive oil
¼ cup fresh basil (chopped)
1½ tbsp. fresh oregano leaves
1 tbsp. ginger juice (fresh)
2 tbsp. lemon juice (fresh)
¼ tsp. unrefined sea salt

Directions:

1. In a food processor or blender, blend cucumber with ginger and lemon juice and olive oil.
2. Then add Brazil nuts to blender and blend until smooth.
3. Remove from blender and place in a bowl.
4. Mix in chopped basil and oregano into dressing.
5. Store in refrigerator in a glass container with a tight fitting lid for up to three days.

Creamy Avocado Dressing

This is a rich, creamy dressing.

Ingredients:
1 avocado
1 clove garlic, freshly minced
½ cucumber, chopped
¼ tsp. unrefined sea salt
½ cup extra virgin organic olive oil
1 tbsp. lime or lemon juice (fresh)

Directions:
1. Combine avocado, garlic, cucumber, lime or lemon juice, and whole, sea salt.
2. Add olive oil in a slow, steady stream while blending the other ingredients together.

Variation:
Substitute balsamic vinegar for lemon juice.

Recipes 3:
Soups

All soups are one to two servings.

Blend them in a blender until smooth.

Enzyme-Rich Spinach Soup

Ingredients:
1 yellow bell pepper (diced)
2 ribs celery (diced)
2 cups baby spinach, minced
1 avocado, peeled, pitted and diced
1 sundried tomato (soaked in water until soft)
1 tbsp. cold-pressed raw flax or hemp seed oil
1 tbsp. cumin
3 tbsp. fresh ground raw pumpkin seeds
5 tbsp. cooked chickpeas, or cooked adzuki beans (mashed)
¼ tsp. unrefined sea salt
1 tbsp. lemon juice, or ½ tbsp. unpasteurized apple cider vinegar
Water, as needed for thinning

Directions:
1. Blend bell pepper, celery, spinach, avocado, soft sundried tomato, cold pressed oil, cumin, lemon or vinegar, and sea salt in a blender until smooth. Add a little pure water to make it thinner if it is too thick.
2. Remove from blender, add the mashed beans, and combine well.
3. Add the freshly ground pumpkin seeds into the mixture.

4. Store in the refrigerator in a glass jar with a tight lid.

Gazpacho

Ingredients:
3 large tomatoes (diced)
1 red, yellow, or orange bell pepper (seeded & diced)
½ cucumber (diced)
¼ cup raw, cold-pressed flax or hemp oil
2 cloves garlic (minced)
2 sundried tomatoes (soaked in pure water until soft)
2 drops of plain liquid stevia
Pinch of black pepper
Pinch of cayenne pepper
Pinch of turmeric
Unrefined sea salt to taste

Directions:
1. Blend all ingredients in a blender until creamy.
2. Serve room temperature or slightly chilled.

Vegetarian Gluten-Free Nutritious Broth

This is a great alkalizing and healing broth. I make it almost weekly and drink it almost daily. Drain off the vegetables and simply drink the broth. Or, you can save the vegetables and eat them separately, or all together as a vegetable soup.

Serving size: 6 servings

Note: Garlic is fragile. Don't cook it too long. You want it to retain as much of its nutritional value as possible.

Ingredients:
1 zucchini (chopped into small chunks with skin)
4 carrots (chopped into small chunks with skin)
3–4 celery stalks (chopped into small pieces)
1 red or sweet onion (chopped into small pieces)
4–5 cloves garlic, minced
1 cup green beans (chopped into small pieces)
2 sweet potatoes (cleaned and chopped into small chunks with skin)
Mineral-rich salt to taste (about 1 tsp.)
Freshly ground pepper to taste
¼ tsp. cumin
5 cups pure, non-chlorinated water

Directions:

1. Place vegetables (cut into chunks), salt, cumin, and pepper in a large pot with the water.
2. Bring to a boil, then turn down and simmer until the potatoes are tender.
3. Add garlic at the end for a few minutes to simmer.
4. Strain off vegetables and drink broth.

Variation:

Substitute (if you have to) frozen vegetables for fresh.

Tzatziki

This Middle Eastern Dip is cool and refreshing on hot summer days. It can be eaten as a soup or a dip with breads, vegetables, and fresh fruit. Serve chilled.

Serving Size: 4 servings.
Note: Leave the peels on the cucumbers for their nutritional benefits.

Ingredients:
2 cups plain or vanilla, raw, unpasteurized, organic goat's milk yogurt
3 small cucumbers, coarsely chopped
2 tbsp. fresh mint leaves
1 clove garlic, minced finely
1 large scallion, peeled and coarsely chopped
2 tbsp. fresh lemon or lime juice
Unrefined sea salt to taste
White pepper to taste

Directions:
1. Place all ingredients in blender or food processor, and puree.

Variations:
Non-pasteurized, Greek-style yogurt works really well in this recipe. You can also use coconut yogurt for this recipe for a dairy-free option.

Recipes 4:
Dip

Hummus

Hummus is a traditional Mediterranean dip that is high in protein and nutrients. It also happens to be very easy to make. I typically make a large batch and continue to eat it all week with different fruits, vegetables, whole grain crackers, or breads. I often use this dip as a creamy sandwich spread. I even refer to myself as the hummus queen, because I like to make it so much and have created numerous variations over the years. This recipe is my favorite.

Ingredients:
3 cups cooked garbanzo beans
1–3 cloves garlic (minced)
5 tbsp. freshly squeezed lemon or lime juice
¼ cup tahini
1 tsp. cumin
1tsp. unrefined sea salt
⅛ tsp. cayenne pepper (optional—Some people don't like the hot taste.)
¼ cup parsley (fresh)

Directions:
1. Combine all ingredients in a food processor and blend until creamy.
2. Serve with cut vegetables crudités as the dipping chips. Examples: sliced cucumber, carrot, celery, crooked neck squash, red or yellow bell pepper, green beans, and zucchini.

Note: Add a little extra-virgin olive oil or coconut oil to the mixture, a little bit at a time, if it's too thick.

Variations: Use other bean varieties, instead of or in addition to the traditional garbanzo bean.

Recipes 5:
Main Dishes

Baked Eggplant

Serving Size: 1 serving

Ingredients:
1 eggplant
Pure, organic coconut oil
Sea salt

Directions:
1. Preheat oven to 350 degrees.
2. Wash the eggplant very well.
3. Slice the eggplant into ¼ inch slices, with the skin.
4. Rub the eggplant with the coconut oil and then sprinkle sea salt on it, both sides. The coconut oil doesn't have to be thick or heavy, just lightly coat it with the coconut oil.
5. Lay the eggplant in a glass or ceramic shallow baking dish.
6. Place the eggplant in the oven for 8–10 minutes, or until the eggplant is soft and warm.
7. Serve warm.

Steamed Vegetables

I like steaming coniferous vegetables because it is better for the thyroid gland.

Ingredients:
Cauliflower, broccoli, yellow neck squash (all cut into bite size pieces)

Directions:
1. Place the cut vegetables in the steamer basket over purified water in a saucepan.
2. Steam just a few minutes, until just barely soft.
3. Sprinkle with a tiny bit of sea salt, or my sensational sea salt seasoning and, if you want, a tiny bit of either coconut oil or ghee.
4. Serve warm.

Basic Stir Fry

Stir frying, or wok cooking, is a healthy way to make a great meal! When you cook, simply keep the foods moving so everything gets heated and cooked without getting overcooked.

This recipe allows you to change the sauce whenever you want to have a new taste sensation. The stir fry can be very light, heart and weight healthy, yet savory and delicious. Mix up the types of vegetables you use and try to buy what's in season. Stir fries are an easy way to have a home-cooked meal without much prep or clean-up time.

Serve this dish warm with a side of sprouted quinoa or sprouted, whole-grain rice, or a bowl of soup.

Ingredients:
2 tbsp. coconut oil
2 cups mushrooms, sliced (button or portabella)
1 tsp. miso
2 tbsp. non-chlorinated water (to mix with miso)
¾ cup (1 large) red onion, chopped
½ cup mushrooms, sliced
½ cup water chestnuts
½ cup snow peas or green beans, cut bite-sized
2 cloves garlic, minced
2 carrots, julienned
1 yellow bell pepper, cored, seeded, cut bite-sized
½ cup water chestnuts or cashews (optional)

Unrefined sea salt and freshly ground black pepper to taste

Directions:
1. Heat oil in stainless steel skillet or wok with chopped red onions for a minute or two.
2. Dissolve miso in 2 tbsp. water, add to the onions, and sauté a brief minute.
3. Add mushrooms and all other ingredients to the pan and stir fry about 6 minutes, constantly stirring and making sure they are cooking evenly and nothing is getting burned.
4. Remove from heat and serve warm.

Variations:
1. Substitute or add some sliced organic, sprouted/cooked lentils or sprouted/cooked beans for the mushrooms.
2. Fresh orange slices taste nice with this dish.
3. Add a little turmeric spice to this stir fry.

Quinoa with Broccoli

Quinoa is gluten-free and is a complete protein. It makes a nice alternative to rice. The darker the variety, the more antioxidants it has. Sprouted quinoa is easier to digest.

Notes:
Add the broccoli over low heat after the quinoa is already cooked. This retains more of the broccoli's nutritional value and live enzymes.

Ingredients:
2 cups quinoa (sprouted)
1 scallion, chopped
4 cups water
½ cup broccoli crowns, cut into bite-sized pieces
¼ cup slivered almonds
1½ tbsp. coconut oil
¼ tsp. sea salt (or add sea salt to taste)

Directions:
1. Place quinoa and all of the white part of the chopped scallion in a pot of water.
2. Cook over medium heat for 15–20 minutes until quinoa is soft.
3. Turn the heat down to low and add broccoli, almonds, remaining scallion, coconut oil, and sea salt. Gently toss for a few moments until

broccoli is a brighter green. Remove from heat quickly.

Note: To sprout quinoa, soak it in pure water overnight and drain off the water before cooking.

Stuffed Red Bell Peppers

Stuffed Red Bell Peppers are a delicious and healthy way to get creative with bell peppers, a vegetable high in antioxidants and Vitamin C. They are a perfect main dish to serve at parties, since you can easily prepare them ahead of time and have them ready to bake. You will need a deep, lidded baking dish that will keep the peppers upright while baking. Each bell pepper will serve one, so adjust the recipe accordingly. Serve warm.

Note: Try to buy peppers that will sit firmly on a flat surface.

Ingredients:
4 red bell peppers, seeds and stems removed, cleaned and halved
3 tbsp. extra-virgin, pure coconut oil
1 sweet onion, finely chopped
2 celery stalks, finely chopped
2 carrots, finely chopped
4 cups sprouted quinoa, cooked (You can buy sprouted quinoa, or you can soak it overnight in non-chlorinated water to remove the phytic acid and make the quinoa healthier. Sprout it before you cook it.)
¼ cup fresh cilantro (or 1 tbsp. dried)
2 tbsp. fresh parsley, chopped
3 tbsp. lemon juice

Unrefined sea salt to taste

Directions:

1. Preheat oven to 375°F.
2. Carefully cut a sliver off the bottom of the peppers, so they will sit upright on a flat surface. Sprinkle peppers lightly with sea salt and set aside.
3. Heat oil in large skillet over medium heat.
4. Add onion, celery, and carrot. Cover and cook until vegetables are softened, approximately five minutes, stirring as needed.
5. Add quinoa, cilantro, parsley, lemon juice, and sea salt. Stir to mix well.
6. Taste and adjust seasonings as needed.
7. Fill the peppers with the sautéed mixture.
8. Stand peppers up in baking dish, and pour ¼ inch water around (not over) the peppers.
9. Cover baking dish with lid.
10. Cook approximately 40–50 minutes, or until peppers are fork-tender.

Recipes 6:
Snacks

Veggies

These fresh veggies make the perfect snack!
- Fresh green beans
- Fresh snow peas
- Fresh okra
- Fresh cucumber
- Fresh celery
- Fresh tomatoes
- Fresh red, yellow, or orange bell pepper

Directions:
1. Buy fresh organic vegetables.
2. Cut off stems and ends.
3. Sprinkle lightly with mineral-rich unrefined sea salt. (This can help you absorb the potassium more effectively.)

You can put washed and cut veggies in individual containers or baggies and put them in the refrigerator for the week. If you crave something a little more filling, have hummus with these veggies as the dipping chips. Or, put a small amount of raw nut or seed butter in the celery.

Fruit

Fresh fruit wedges or fresh berries are a healthy and delicious snack.

- Orange
- Grapefruit
- Tangerine
- Berries
- Cherries
- Papaya
- Mango
- Apple
- Pear
- Bananas

Consume fruit by itself. Always eat the whole fresh fruit. Never drink pure fruit juice, because it is too high in natural sugar. It's better to eat the whole fresh fruit with the fiber. Try to consume tree-ripened fruit, because it has natural immune system boosters.

I would say to avoid bananas because most of the calories in bananas come from carbohydrates, with 34 grams per cup. According to the MayoClinic.com, low-carb diets can help with weight loss by lowering your levels of insulin, which potentially helps you burn fat.

But there are a few ways I would say you can eat bananas. If you have a craving for ice cream, a great way to satisfy that craving and avoid high-sugar ice cream is to freeze bananas and eat small bites of banana instead of ice cream. They are delicious frozen, and you can eat a few bites and avoid consuming something that is not as healthy.

Another way you could use bananas in a healthy way is in a smoothie. If you do use a banana, make sure it's really clean, cut off the ends, and put the entire banana (with the fiber and nutrient-dense skin on it) in a blender. It tastes just the same, but has the added nutrition and fiber. The banana skin has more nutrients in it than the fruit itself. The fiber and antioxidants in the skin can help support your adrenal glands.

Lightly adding some mineral rich salt or my sensational sea salt seasoning can help your body absorb potassium optimally.

14
Fresh Produce Storage Tips

Fresh produce is part of this healthy eating plan and lifestyle. Storing it properly is important. We go to the store and buy delicious-looking food. But then we get home and end up storing it improperly, or we get busy and forget about it. Then we find our refrigerator having the aroma of over-ripe or rotting fruits and veggies. One way we can spend less AND eat healthier is by storing our fresh food properly.

Many times, we go to the store and see all the beautiful fresh fruits and veggies in season and on sale, and we over buy. So, first try to only buy what you truly feel you are going to eat in the next few days. Don't try to buy produce to last for a week. It may not last that long. Some root veggies can last a month, if stored properly, but fresher, more fragile fruits and veggies will only last about 2 -5 days. If you do buy too much, you can think about making a pie, or doing some canning, or freezing some of your more fragile fruits and veggies before they spoil.

Always store your food in its complete wholeness. According to food scientist Barry Swanson at Washington State University, if you pull fruits and vegetables apart, you have broken the cells, and microorganisms will immediately begin to grow. So, avoid breaking the skin and leave the stem intact. He also says you should never place fruits and veggies in airtight bags. That actually will speed up the decay. You do want to be mindful that mold will proliferate quickly and can spoil the whole group of fruits or veggies. So, toss out any spoiled produce immediately, or put it into your compost bin.

Next, make sure you are storing the various types of fruits and veggies with the right partners. Some give off high levels of ethylene gas (a ripening agent), which makes them and everything around them ripen or decay quickly. You want to keep these types of foods separate from each other. Put things like kale and spinach in the same bin, and peaches and apples in another. If you put fruit with greens, it will cause the greens to rot or turn yellow in a few days. Greens are very sensitive to the ethylene gas. I have a little product called an E.G.G. (Ethylene Gas Guardian, which is shaped like an egg), and it absorbs the ethylene. I just put it in my bin with the fruits and/or greens. Of course, if you need something to ripen faster, then you can use this knowledge to your advantage. You can put the one you need to ripen with a fruit that gives off the high level of ethylene gas. I also use produce bags by Bio-Fresh and Evert-Fresh. They will absorb ethylene gas and help your produce stay fresher longer.

Keep root veggies (including all kinds of potatoes) in a cool, dark, dry place. They can last up to a month if kept properly. Never store potatoes in the refrigerator, because they will develop much higher sugar content.

Here is a list of fruits and veggies, showing the best way to store them. These are high ethylene producers, and you can refrigerate them: apples, apricots, avocados, blueberries, cantaloupe, cherimoyas, cranberries, figs, green onions, guavas, grapes, honeydew, kiwifruit, mangoes, nectarines, papayas, passion fruit, peaches, pears, persimmons, plums, prunes, quince, and tomatoes.

A banana is a high releaser but should be stored in a cool dark place outside of the refrigerator.

These are very sensitive to ethylene gas: asparagus, bananas (unripe), blackberries, broccoli, Brussels sprouts, cabbage, carrots, cauliflower, chard, cucumbers, eggplant, endive, garlic, green beans, kale, leafy greens, leeks, lettuce, okra, onions, parsley, peas, peppers, raspberries, spinach, squash, strawberries, watercress, and watermelon. Keep them separate from the high ethylene gas producing foods.

Mushrooms should be stored in a dry paper bag or breathable container and put in a cool place. I've been told to gently brush them off under water to clean them before preparing them for consumption.

Try to purchase fresh fruits and veggies that have been ripened on the vine or on the tree. Tree or vine-ripened foods contain salvestrols, which are compounds that have natural anti-cancer properties.[30] In fact, the word salvestrol comes from the Latin word "save." So, growing your own food or buying from a local farmer is one way of getting food that is vine or tree-ripened. Food that is picked green and then ripened on the way to market does not contain these salvestrols.

Organic food is best, because it is more nutrient dense. Chemical fertilizers and pesticides can destroy nutrients in the soil, like sulfur and chromium, which are vital for our health. "The Organic Center study found that organic foods were more nutritionally dense in 61% of the cases" and they "found conventional foods to contain higher nitrates, which are widely considered a potential health hazard."[31]

With all the fresh fruits and vegetables enticing us from their bins at the farmer's market or grocery store, now we can make those delicious meals with our properly stored produce!

Bon Appétit!

15
Travel Tips

E ating healthy while traveling can be very challenging. Here are some helpful ideas. When ordering food at a restaurant, ask for the oil and vinegar to be brought to the table so you can make your own dressing. This way, you can be sure it doesn't have additives like sugar or MSG or sulfites in it.

Take your own food with you for emergencies.

I have raw food bars from the Garden of Life, including a raw green bar with chocolate coating and a berry bar I take with me when traveling. This way, I do not risk getting so hungry that I buy something terrible for me. I know these bars are good for me, and will satisfy my hunger and sustain me for a fairly long time.

Another thing I take is Garden of Life protein powder mix and their green food powder, Perfect Food (cacao flavor), in a baggie or container with a small spoon. It easily mixes with water. It is vegan, raw, organic, non-GMO, and nutrient dense. I can easily mix this up (even with water) and drink it almost any time or place.

I also take a few tea bags with me, my little portable bottle of stevia, and my whole, unrefined sea salt with me. These are my staples when I travel. I am hardly ever without them, even in town.

At restaurants, I order off the side dish or appetizer menu. When deciding whether to order steamed veggies or slightly sautéed veggies, I ask about what fat they sauté them in. I order steamed if it is a fat I don't approve of. Avoid all-you-can-eat buffets! They are very rough on someone wanting to eat smaller portions.

When I buy purified water, I always add my unrefined sea salt to it. This puts electrolytes in my water, and I can hydrate more efficiently. I also make sure I drink half my weight in ounces of water a day. I weigh about 100 lbs., so I drink 50 oz. of water every day. Drinking plenty of water keeps me from getting too dehydrated on the road.

16
Joint, Tissue, and Skin Health

This chapter doesn't directly address weight loss, but I've found that many people who have struggled with weight loss or aging have painful joints or problems with saggy, thin, wrinkly skin. So, I wanted to share with you about a supplement I take. Liquid Biocell is a supplement that has helped me immensely with joint and back pain. It has also helped me with my skin thickness and hydration. I thought I would share this with you.

I'm using a fairly new hyaluronic acid and collagen supplement. This revolutionary product is an exclusive, award-winning, multi-patented formula that includes antioxidant-rich super fruits and Resveratrol, all in a delicious, liquid dietary supplement. The combination of these ingredients works synergistically to promote healthy aging, active joints, and younger-looking skin.

This cellular support product is a multi-patented joint and skin health nutraceutical that contains a naturally occurring matrix of hyaluronic acid, chondroitin sulfate, and hydrolyzed collagen. It has been the subject of several clinical studies which demonstrated its safety and efficacy. Unlike ordinary dietary supplements containing a blend of multiple ingredients, this matrix is made from a single naturally occurring source and utilizes an international, multi-patented process which ensures rapid absorption. It is totally drug-free with no known side effects. It has also been approved by the National Sports Federation (NSF) for use by athletes for endurance and recovery, as well as joint health.

Canada researched the clinical trials of this supplement. Because of their findings, Canada requires the company to place this information about this product on the label: "Helps to relieve joint pain associated with osteoarthritis of the hip and knee. Helps to maintain healthy skin. Helps the body to metabolize fats and proteins. Helps in the development and maintenance of bones, cartilage, teeth and gums. Helps in connective tissue formation. Helps in wound healing. An antioxidant for the maintenance of good health."

I feel like it is a "fountain of youth" supplement. I had severe back and hip pain as a result of scoliosis. I thought I'd have to live with it, and I didn't want to do the suggested surgery. I have been taking this supplement since January, 2014, and I no longer have back or hip pain. It is truly great, living free of that pain. In addition, people are saying my skin is looking fantastic. They are even asking me if I got a facelift, which I have not.

This product reduces wrinkles from the inside out, naturally!

I've also had some of my clients take it. They have had equally good success with their joint pain when they commit to it and stick with it long enough for it to supplement what's been depleted in their body. I always recommend the 90-day challenge. You need to give it time to work and replenish your body.

If you want to take your health to a new, cellular level, I will help you place your first order and answer any questions you have. Use the following web address and get $10 off:

http://www.modere.com/?referralCode=j220555

There are also equine and pet versions, which work extraordinarily well. To learn more, email me: Nancy@organichealthylifestyle.com.

17
Easy Ways to Make Healthy Eating Delicious!

I frequently talk to people who think that eating healthier doesn't always taste delicious. But the good news is that when we start doing something new, our bodies adapt and our taste buds acclimate. When you change your diet and start eating a different type of food, it may not initially seem quite as delicious as you hoped it would. That's because you have not been eating that food until now, and your taste buds are not used to it. But, if you continue to eat that specific food on a continual basis for about two weeks, your body will adapt and your taste buds will generate and acclimate to these new taste sensations. Stick with the new, healthier diet and allow your body to grow and evolve with you. Within two weeks, that new food will taste better than it did the first time.

So, let's get started on a new eating plan for a healthier, happier you! To begin this new dietary journey, get a fresh start with seven of my top tips for making healthy eating delicious!

One: Use healthy fat in your recipes. Eating fat does not necessarily make a person fat. In fact, the right kinds of fat can make people skinny, as well as support overall health and increase energy.

The advertising industry would have us believe that fat is bad or fattening. But in reality, good fat can be critical to our health and our weight management. Fat actually tells the body how to utilize protein and carbohydrates. Fat in our food can make it taste rich and satisfying. Foods that are savory usually have some fat in them, but many low-fat or fat-free products are filled with salt, sugar, chemical additives, and MSG to make up for the lack of savory flavor the fat provides.

Coconut oil and avocado oil are examples of pure, unprocessed healthy fats. Coconut oil is seen in most parts of the world as the super-food of fats. Coconut oil is a healthy "nut" fat. It is a highly chemically stable fat, meaning it can be heated without negative effects. Very few oils handle heat well, but certain coconut oils handle high heat very well. It is also resistant to lipid peroxidation (which may be a common mechanistic pathway that can lead to increased cancer risk)[32] and rancidity.

Coconut oil is unique if you are a calorie counter. Coconut oil has 2.6% fewer calories per gram than other fats. Coconut oil nourishes the body, and its medium-chained fatty acids provide a good source of energy. Coconut oil is also highly effective as an antioxidant.

Coconut oil is a safe alternative oil for any cooking recipe. And as a healthy fat, it makes food taste rich and savory!

Avocados are a superfood filled with vitamins, minerals, and healthy fat. They are especially high in potassium and fiber, which contribute to weight loss and have been linked to a lower risk of disease.

Two: Use mushrooms in your recipes. Studies show mushrooms aid the immune system because they are rich in potassium, selenium, copper, riboflavin, niacin, and pantothenic acid, and B complex vitamins. Some kinds of mushrooms are one of only two natural food sources of Vitamin D. Mushrooms are an excellent source of the antioxidants polyphenols, selenium, and ergothioneine (known as a master antioxidant, an amino acid containing sulfur. Sulfur is an extremely important nutrient, yet it is highly overlooked.) One medium portobello mushroom has more potassium than a small banana. Five medium cremini mushrooms have more selenium than a large egg or three ounces of lean beef. Plus, the copper in mushrooms helps the body to make red blood cells, which carry oxygen throughout the body.

Mushrooms are low in calories and are about 80–90% water, which makes them a great substitute for meat in recipes when wanting to cut calories. Studies also show that consuming mushrooms daily can help prevent cancer by up to 64%.[33] (Both fresh and dried mushrooms were found to work, but the fresh mushrooms worked better.)

Adding mushrooms to dishes is easy. Thinly slice some mushrooms and put them on salads, pasta dishes, and sandwiches—or serve them as a side dish. Grilling them is always great, and mushrooms make a tasty and healthy alternative to a burger. I love to sauté them with onions and butter in order to bring out the rich flavor of savory mushrooms. Each mushroom has a different flavor, so experiment by trying different varieties.

Three: Eat colorful, fresh, organic food to get antioxidants. Antioxidants are in the color. Avoid white, refined foods and choose the ones with rich color. For example, in the winter, certain seasonal foods like root vegetables can be very comforting, especially potatoes! But instead of white potatoes, give yourself an antioxidant boost by trying red potatoes, purple potatoes, yams, or sweet potatoes. Sweet potatoes are delicious, and high in fiber and beta-carotene.

Use coconut oil as a healthy fat in potato dishes. Mix it in to mashed potatoes, or use it when you cut potatoes up for baking and frying. If you want a buttery flavor, add a tiny bit of ghee to the coconut oil. Just remember: Never store potatoes in the refrigerator. Doing this will turn the starch in potatoes into sugar.

Four: Cook with unrefined sea salt to increase your health and well-being. When I ask people if they use salt, they usually tell me, "No, I eat a low-salt diet for health reasons." But unrefined sea salt is not salt that is bad for us. It is the type of salt we eat that dictates whether it is good for you.

The word "electrolyte" is a fancy medical term for salt. We need electrolytes to be healthy. Our immune systems can't function without them. In fact, low-salt diets promote toxicity, and they have adverse effects on the body. Low-salt diets promote elevated insulin levels and insulin resistance, as well as elevated normal cholesterol and LDL cholesterol levels. Low-salt diets will lead to mineral deficiencies and the development of chronic disease.

Adding unrefined, mineral rich sea salt to your diet can increase the usable oxygen in your blood, detoxify blood, and neutralize radiation. Unrefined, mineral-rich sea salt makes capillaries more elastic and increases blood flow. There are various types of unrefined sea salt, all containing different mineral contents. Try a few different ones and see which you like the best.

Five: Add spices to your food to add flavor and incredible health benefits. Two spices I most recommend adding are turmeric and cinnamon. Turmeric is a common ingredient in Indian cuisine and contains an ingredient called curcumin. Curcumin has more than 150 therapeutic agents to combat viruses, bacterium, diseases, and other chronic conditions. Turmeric can help curb indigestion and heartburn. It protects brain and cardiovascular health, boosts the immune system and decreases inflammation. Turmeric works better when combined with fat and if you combine it with black pepper, you can increase the rate of absorption 1000 times.

Ceylon Cinnamon is another spice you can add to your recipes. It us very effective in lowering blood sugar levels.[34]

Six: Use healthier sweeteners. Sugar is like an addictive drug. It gives the body an artificial energy surge, and the body begins to crave that energy. Dr. Francis Stern states, "A characteristic of sugar 'binges' is that the taste for sweets, for some reason, leads to a craving for more of the same, just the way other drugs create cravings."[35] I encourage you to limit or eliminate sugar from your diet as much as possible. A few suggestions for when you wish to add a sweetener are honey, xylitol, dates or date sugar.

Honey is a natural sweetener that is antifungal and antibacterial. Honey contains a variety of nutrients and minerals, as well as some enzymes. It is known to facilitate muscle recuperation and glycogen restoration after a workout. Substitute honey for sugar in recipes. Always buy raw, unrefined honey so that live enzymes and nutritional properties are still intact.

Xylitol is a sugar alcohol found in fruits and vegetables. It is made from birch tree bark and other hard wood trees. Xylitol has fewer calories and 75% fewer carbohydrates than sugar. Studies have shown that ingesting xylitol can alkalize your body, reduce sugar cravings, and reduce insulin levels. It was approved by the FDA in 1963. (Note: *Xylitol is toxic to pets.*)

Seven: Use delicious probiotic foods in your recipes. Probiotic food is vital to the health and strength of the immune system, and it supports digestion and absorption of food and nutrients. Adding garlic, onions, raw, unprocessed apple cider vinegar, raw, unprocessed soy sauce, coconut yogurts, kombucha, and miso to your recipes can make them delicious as well as create a healthier immune system!

Allium vegetables, like garlic and onions, have been studied extensively in relation to cancer. Their beneficial and preventative effects are likely due in part to their rich organosulfur compounds. Garlic, in particular, has a wonderful flavor. It's fragile, so I add it at the end of cooking. Adding onion is a great way to add flavor to a dish without adding extra calories. Onions can be sautéed, roasted, and grilled or caramelized. Use them fresh as a topping for sandwiches or salads, or add them to salsas and dips. They have both probiotic and antifungal properties.

Fermented foods are foods that have been through a process of lactofermentation, in which natural bacteria feed on the sugar in the food to create lactic acid. This process preserves the food. It creates beneficial enzymes, B vitamins,

So, lighten up, get going, and embrace a new, healthier lifestyle! By incorporating delicious, healthier ingredients into your recipes you will give your body some necessary tools to help it heal and stay healthier in the future. Now is the time to transition to a healthier lifestyle that you can maintain for the rest of your life! Feel lighter and brighter in your body, mind, and spirit.

It's time for new adventures with food!

18
A Closing Note

Writing this book has been a joy for me. I have learned so much over the years and now find so much happiness in being able to share all of this information with you. May you find health and happiness with the healthier lifestyle you are embracing. Bless you.

And remember:
The Main Ingredient is Always Love!

For more great recipes and nutrition information, see my best-selling, award-winning books *How to Be a Healthy Vegetarian (Second Edition)* and *Diabetes and Your Diet*, both of which are half cookbook and half nutrition/lifestyle information.

How to Be a Healthy Vegetarian:
myBook.to/vegetarianbook

Diabetes and Your Diet:
myBook.to/diabetesandyourdiet

To sign up for my free monthly newsletter, visit
www.OrganicHealthyLife.com

Dedication and Acknowledgments

First and foremost, I thank God for the constant love, support, inspiration, knowledge, experiences, and energy that it took to put this book together. May God bless this book and all who read it.

Heartfelt thanks and dedication to my children: *Amanda Gibbons Addison* and *Frederick Gibbons Addison*. You are the loves of my life and my biggest fans, and I am yours. As my original taste-testers, you helped me prepare, develop, refine, and taste-test all of my new ideas all of your lives. My heart overflows with love for you. Thank you for a lifetime of your unwavering support and love.

Thank you to my mother Junia Gibbons, my sister Jane, her husband David, their child Claire and her husband Stefan, and their children Audrey and Reid. Thank you to my sister Liz, her husband Layne, and their children: Jack and his wife Amber, and their children Annie, Mary and Ford; Clayton and his wife Lynsie, and their child Scout. Thanks to my brother Patrick and his son Ryan; to my sister Mary, her husband Rusty, and their children, Carter, Katie, and Rebecca. Your love and support for my children and me has been a godsend. You enrich my life every day. I'm so fortunate to be a part of this family.

Thank you to my precious daughter-in-law Edy and her wonderful parents Chip and Cynthia Jones. I am honored with your love, generosity, encouragement, friendship, and support. I love your family, and I am thrilled to share my son with you.

An enormous thank you to Dr. Sandra Bontemps for the thoughtful and kind contribution of the foreword. I also want to thank you for your friendship and consistent encouragement.

A great big thank you to Dr. Gary Massad for his consistent faith, support, and encouragement.

To all of the wonderful friends and neighbors from my life who have honored me with their friendship, never-ending patience, cheerful words of encouragement, and constant support, I thank you all for making my life so much brighter. Bless you all.

Thank you to all of my friends and associates at Allie Beth Allman and Associates for your kindness, generosity, and encouragement. Also thanks to all of my friends from Highland Park for your encouragement, faith, and friendship through the years.

Thank you to my dear friend Lisa Endicott of Lisa Endicott PR and staff for all you have done for me with skill, expertise, thoughtfulness, and kind consideration. You have been there with me throughout all my journeys. You've enriched my life, and it has been a delight to work with you.

A special thank you to Susan Doyle, Cindy Williams, Deanna Sweet, James Wynne, Maryann De Leo, Roy Teeluck, Linda Gray, Grimanes Amoras, Adele Good, Stephanie Askew, Mark Pharo, Charlotte Ammerman, Kirk Dooley, Michael Reisman, Dr. Bill Osmunson, DDS, Nick Sakulenzki, Kelley Willis, Priscilla Miller, Janneth Whitworth , Julianne Parker, Eve Baughman Yung, Suann Davis, Dr. Therese Rowley, Densil Adams, Kimberly Wechsler, Alan Rodriguez, Earl Rector, Susan Staples, Susan Williams, Karis Adams, Trish Aldredge, Kurt Boxdorfer, Dr. Anitra Thorhaug, Julie Goss, Judd Walker, Lori Markman, Mary Monttein Alonso, Debbie Russell, Nancy Miller, Mary Jo Rausch, Kathleen Hayden, Richard Kemp, Andrea and Randy Harrah, Harrison Evans, Chris Koustoubardis, Prudie and Rick Koeninger, Marilyn Flemming, Candace Stone, Becky Crow Nolan, Jacqueline Cornaby, Orvel Ray Wilson, Gina Carr, Tim Durkin, Dave Lieber and so many friends who have helped me in more ways than I can list.

Thank you to my Health Nuts Group: Sheila Fitzgerald, Dr. Mary Warren, Dr. Elizabeth Naylor, Dean Vanderslice and Denise Ringer. It has been a fun and interesting journey with you.

Thanks to all of my dear friends at the National Speakers Association and the north Texas chapter for all your help, support, kindness, and generosity. I am very grateful for you. A warm thank you to Dr. Jan Goss for believing in me. Thank you for your support and continued encouragement.

A huge thank you to Matthew Howard for helping me edit and design this book.

Thank you to Lori Brennan and Kytka Hilmar-Jezek for my cover design, and so much more!

I am grateful for all of you. Bless you all. Please accept my deepest, heartfelt thanks.

About the Author

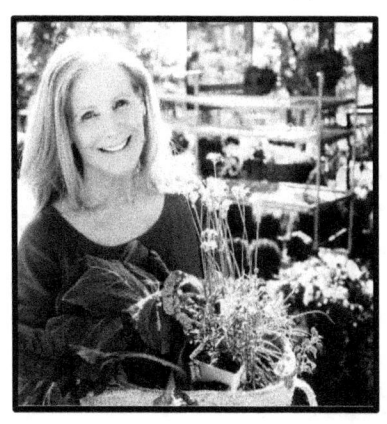

Nancy is the number one best-selling author of *Raising Healthy Children*, *How to Be a Healthy Vegetarian* (first and second editions), and co-author of *Alive & Cooking: An Easy Guide to Health for You and Your Parents*. Nancy is a health counselor, certified by Columbia University and the Institute of Integrative Nutrition. Nancy specializes in eating disorders, asthma, diabetes, heart disease, arthritis/joint problems, and weight loss. Nancy holds a Certificate for Plant-Based Nutrition from Cornell University and the T. Colin Campbell Foundation, and is a board-certified health practitioner with the American Association of Drugless Practitioners. She studied with Natalia Rose and the Rose Program in Detoxification, and is a certified raw food chef, instructor, and teacher with Alissa Cohen. Nancy is certified in Basic Intensive in Health—Supportive Cooking from the Natural Gourmet Institute for Food & Health in

New York. Nancy is certified in sports nutrition and is a certified personal trainer.

Nancy is the health, food, and recipe columnist for *Celebration Magazine*. She is a member of the National Speakers Association and Global Speakers Federation. She studied at the Mediterranean Cooking School in Syros, Greece, and the Australasian College of Health Science. She studied conscious farming (organic gardening) at the Tree of Life Rejuvenation Center with John M. Phillips of the Living Earth Training Center. Nancy holds a Bachelor of Arts degree from Hollins College (now University) in Roanoke, Virginia, and a lifelong Texas teaching certificate for all grade levels. She is a certified licensed wildlife rehabilitator. She studied at Le Cordon Bleu culinary school in London, England. Nancy also served as secretary of the Earth Society, an affiliate of the United Nations. Nancy is a certified practitioner of psychosomatic therapy.

Nancy's delightful celebration of healthy food and her passion for sharing her wealth of knowledge is entertaining, enlightening, and, many times, life changing. Through presentations and counseling, Nancy shares her favorite tips for getting healthier and making healthy eating delicious. Nancy's information-packed books and presentations are inspiring, and her joy contagious! You will learn how to celebrate life by living a healthier lifestyle.

Contact Nancy if you would like personal
counseling: Nancy@OrganicHealthyLifestyle.com

- Listen to Nancy's radio show on I Heart Radio:
  http://www.iheart.com/show/209-Organic-
  Healthy-Lifestyle/?episode_id=27165830
- Sign up for Nancy's free monthly newsletter:
  www.OrganicHealthyLifestyle.com
- Visit Nancy on Facebook:
  www.facebook.com/authornancyaddison

Recommended Companies and Products

Blue Mountain Organics for organic sprouted seeds, nuts, nut and seed butters, sprouted flours, and more.
https://www.bluemountainorganics.com

Rose Mountain Herbs for teas, aromatherapy, foods, essential oils, and more.
https://www.mountainroseherbs.com/#AID=136219

NYR Organics for certified organic make-up, body care, baby care, essential oils, and more.
https://us.nyrorganic.com/shop/nancyaddison_1

Liquid Biocell: This is what I take for joint health, healing properties, and skin health. I love it! I feel like this is my fountain of youth supplement! Contact me if you would like me to help you order it. This is a fantastic company and product. There are pet and equine versions, too.
https://www.modere.com/?referralCode=j220555

Spring Aqua: This is the best water system for the home. It cleans it, mineralizes it, infuses it with hydrogen, and structures it. This is what I bought for my home.
https://water.springaqua.com/nancyaddison

Or call Kenny Lu and tell him Nancy sent you. (206) 913-8888.

Young Living Oils mouthwash. https://www.youngliving.com/us/en/referral/289 856

Institute of Integrative Nutrition (IIN) for a free download of healthy recipes. https://www.integrativenutrition.com/iin-book-download?erefer=0015000000IyQPEAA3

Contact Nancy@OrganicHealthyLifestyle.com if you have any questions.

Notes

[1] Smith, Jeffrey M. (September, 2013). "Can Genetically-Engineered Foods Explain the Exploding Gluten Sensitivity?" *Institute for Responsible Technology.* http://responsibletechnology.org/media/images/content/Exploding-Gluten-Sensitivity_.pdf

[2] Bassler, Dr. Anthony. (2004, January). "A Common Mistake that Prevents Most People from Losing Weight...and How to Avoid It! Why This Simple 'First Step' Should Be Part of Any Weight Management, Anti-Aging and Health Improvement Program." *Vegetarian Times.*

[3] Jensen, Bernard. (1980). *Tissue Cleansing Through Bowel Management.* Escondido, CA: self-published.

[4] Anderson, Richard. "Colon Plaque - Mucoid Plaque." *Cleanse.net.* http://cleanse.net/mucoid-plaque
Dr. Richard Anderson, ND, NMD, is the author of *Cleanse and Purify* Yourself (Avery Trade, revised edition 1998).

[5] Yerba Prima. *Kalenite pill product website.* http://www.yerba.com/index.php?s=kalenite

[6] Mercola, Dr. Joseph. "Here's the Smarter Oil Alternative I Recommend to Replace Those Other Oils in Your Kitchen." *Dr. Mercola Premium Products.* http://products.mercola.com/coconut-oil/

[7] Aglaée Jacob, MS, RD, CDE. (October, 2013). Coconut oil: learn more about this superfood that contains healthful saturated fats. *Today's Dietitian*, 15(10):56. http://www.todaysdietitian.com/newarchives/100713p56.shtml

[8] Nagao, K, and Yanagita, T. (2010). Medium-chain fatty acids: Functional lipids for the prevention and treatment of the metabolic syndrome. *Pharmacological Research*, 61(3):208-212. Retrieved from http://www.meltorganic.com/wp-content/uploads/2011/06/Medium-chain-fatty-acids-Functional-lipids-for-the-prevention-and-treatment-of-the-metabolic-syndrome.pdf

⁹ Assunção, ML, et. al. (July, 2009). Effects of dietary coconut oil on the biochemical and anthropometric profiles of women presenting abdominal obesity. *Lipids*, 44(7):593-601. DOI:10.1007/s11745-009-3306-6.

¹⁰ Johnson, Lorie. (Jan. 05, 2012). "Coconut Oil Touted as Alzheimer's Remedy." *The Christian Broadcasting Network.* www.cbn.com/cbnnews/healthscience/2012/January/Coconut -Oil-Touted-as-Alzheimers-Remedy/

¹¹ Christmas, Ellsworth P., Hawkins, Stephen S. Winter. "Canola: An Alternative Crop in Indiana." *Department of Agronomy, Purdue University.* https://www.extension.purdue.edu/extmedia/AY/AY-272.html

¹² Weigel, Jen. (July 20, 2009). "Healthy Eating with a Spiritual Twist." *Chicago Now.* www.chicagonow.com/blogs/spiritual-dammit/2009/07/healthy-eating-with-a-spiritual-twist.html#ixzz1S8wMYSoL

¹³ Linos, Athena, et. al. (December, 1999). Dietary factors in relation to rheumatoid arthritis: a role for olive oil and cooked vegetables? *The American Journal of Clinical Nutrition*, 70(6):1077-1082. Abstract retrieved from http://ajcn.nutrition.org/content/70/6/1077.short

¹⁴ Tandel, Kirtida R. (Oct-Dec, 2011). Sugar substitutes: health controversy over perceived benefits." *Journal of Pharmacology & Pharmacotherapeutics*, 2(4): 236–243. http://www.ncbi.nlm.nih.gov/pmc/articles/PMC3198517/

¹⁵ MedlinePlus. "Methanol Poisoning." http://www.nlm.nih.gov/medlineplus/ency/article/002680.htm

¹⁶ Gold, Mark. (January, 2003). *Recall aspartame as a neurotoxic drug: file #4: reported aspartame toxicity reactions.* http://www.fda.gov/ohrms/dockets/dailys/03/jan03/012203/02p-0317_emc-000199.txt

¹⁷ Ibid.

¹⁸ Brownstein, David. (2012). *Salt Your Way to Health*, p. 17. 2nd edition. West Bloomfield, MI: Medical Alternative Press.

¹⁹ Ibid., pp. 120,107, 87.

²⁰ Ibid, p. 26.

21 Ibid., p. 53.

22 Geleijnse, J.M., et. al. (1994, August 13). "Reduction in Blood Pressure with a Low Sodium, High Potassium, High Magnesium Salt in Older Subjects with Mild to Moderate Hypertension." *British Medical Journal*, 309, 436–40. http://www.bmj.com/content/309/6952/436

23 Brown University. "Being a Vegetarian." http://brown.edu/Student_Services/Health_Services/Health_ Education/nutrition_&_eating_concerns/being_a_vegetarian. php#4

24 ADA. (2009). Position of the American Dietetic Association. *Journal of the American Dietetic Association*, 109:1266-1282. http://www.vrg.org/nutrition/2009_ADA_position_paper.pdf

25 Esselstyn, Jr., Dr. Caldwell B. (2008). *Prevent and Reverse Heart Disease: The Revolutionary, Scientifically Proven, Nutrition-Based Cure*. New York, New York: Penguin.

26 McDougall, MD, John. "Nutrition in the Medical Clinic Part III" lecture. "Plant-Based Nutrition." eCornell University.

27 Campbell, T. Colin. "Principles of Nutritional Health" lecture. "Plant-Based Nutrition." eCornell University and the T. Colin Campbell Foundation. 2010.

28 Yokoyama, Y., et al. (October, 2014). Vegetarian diets and glycemic control in diabetes: A systematic review and meta-analysis. Cardiovascular Diagnosis & Therapy, 4(5):373–382. DOI: 10.3978/j.issn.2223-3652.2014.10.04. http://www.thecdt.org/article/view/4977/5858

30 Johnson, Dr. Ben. Qtd. in Bollinger, Ty. (2014). *The quest for the cures... continues*. (Film transcript). TTAC Publishing.

31 Steury, Tim. (Winter, 2009). "Is organic more nutritious?" *Washington State Magazine*. http://wsm.wsu.edu/s/index.php?id=749

32 Gago-Dominguez, Manuela, et. al. (2007). Lipid peroxidation, oxidative stress genes and dietary factors in breast cancer protection: a hypothesis. *Breast Cancer Research* 2006, 9:201. http://www.breast-cancer-research.com/content/9/1/201

33 "Eating mushrooms daily 'may cut breast cancer risk by two thirds'." (16 March, 2009). *The Telegraph*. http://www.telegraph.co.uk/news/health/news/5000582/Eati

ng-mushrooms-daily-may-cut-breast-cancer-risk-by-two-thirds.html

[34] "Cinnamon's Health Benefits: Wondering how to lower blood sugar? Try some cinnamon, which has double duty benefits." (2007, November 7.) *Women'sHealth.* http://www.womenshealthmag.com/food/cinnamon-benefits-explained

[35] Goulart, Frances Sheridan. (1991, March 1). "Are You Sugar Smart? Linked to Heart Attacks, Kidney Disease, Diabetes and Other Diseases, Sugar Is to the '90s What Cholesterol Was to the '80s (Includes 9 ways to Cope with Sugar Cravings)." *American Fitness.* http://www.highbeam.com/doc/1G1-10722552.html